Dancing among the Maenads

The Reshaping of Psychoanalysis
From Sigmund Freud to Ernest Becker

Barry R. Arnold
General Editor
Vol. 5

Kevin Volkan

Dancing among the Maenads

The Psychology
of Compulsive Drug Use

PETER LANG
New York • Washington, D.C./Baltimore • San Francisco
Bern • Frankfurt am Main • Berlin • Vienna • Paris

Library of Congress Cataloging-in-Publication Data

Volkan, Kevin.
   Dancing among the maenads: the psychology of compulsive drug use /
by Kevin Volkan.
      p.   cm. — (The Reshaping of psychoanalysis: vol. 5)
    Includes bibliographical references and indexes.
    1. Substance abuse—Psychological aspects. 2. Drug abuse—
Psychological aspects. 3. Psychoanalysis. I. Title. II. Series.
    [DNLM: 1. Substance Abuse—psychology 2. Substance
Dependence—psychology 3. Object Attachment. WM 270 V916d 1994]
RC564.V65   1994   616.86′001′9—dc20   93-23071
DNLM/DLC   CIP
for Library of Congress
ISBN 0-8204-2301-7
ISSN 1059-3551

Die Deutsche Bibliothek-CIP-Einheitsaufnahme

Volkan, Kevin:
Dancing among the maenads: the psychology of compulsive drug use / Kevin
Volkan. - New York; San Francisco; Bern; Baltimore; Frankfurt am Main;
Berlin; Wien; Paris: Lang, 1994
   (The reshaping of psychoanalysis; Vol. 5)
   ISBN 0-8204-2301-7
NE: GT

Cover design by James F. Brisson.

The paper in this book meets the guidelines for permanence and durability of
the Committee on Production Guidelines for Book Longevity of the
Council on Library Resources.

© Peter Lang Publishing, Inc., New York 1994

Printed in the United States of America.

For Jimi Hendrix, who despite his troubles, gave us so much beauty, joy, and truth.

Foreword

Psychoanalytic theories of compulsive drug use, or drug addiction have evolved in concert with psychoanalytic theory in general and reflect the growth, changes, deviations and controversies in the field. Although I did not write this book with the history of psychoanalysis in mind, the historical perspective has informed my understanding of compulsive drug use, just as the study of compulsive drug use has informed my understanding of the history of psychoanalysis. These two viewpoints are really indispensable to one another, and together, paint a picture of psychoanalysis as it has developed over the years. It is my hope that the reader will derive a taste of the theoretical complexity spawned by Freud's seminal insights on compulsive drug use.

The most difficult thing about writing a book about drug use has been to try and remain apolitical. By not taking a political stand (or not sharing my convictions with the reader), I am hoping to reach a wider audience. Nevertheless, it would be unfair to the reader to let my negative bias towards the current status (both legal and cultural) of drugs remain unknown, as it has at least unconsciously influenced my writing. It is my desire, however, not to alienate anyone on a particular side of the drug use debate and, therefore, I have tried to remain as neutral as possible throughout the book. Others scholars, most notably Thomas Sazsz (1992), have taken the opposite approach, taking a strong stand for their political positions. While I most heartily applaud this strength of conviction, I would prefer that my readers draw their own conclusions. I, therefore, ask the reader to excuse any bias in the text, think for him or her self, and form independent opinions on the issues related to the use of drugs.

Acknowledgments

It goes without saying that this work could not have been completed without help from colleagues, family and friends. First, I would like to thank my wife, Panda Kroll, M.F.A. for her editing, expert typesetting and loving criticism. I would also like to thank my father, Vamik Volkan, M.D. for his expert editing and encouragement. Professors Geoffrey Pullum, Ph.D. and James Gill, Ph.D., while serving as Deans of the Graduate School at U.C. Santa Cruz, valued my scholarly aspirations enough to allow me to work part-time while I was writing this book. Kerstin Goldsmith and Laura McEntee brought me joy, friendship and a touch of youthful energy during the creation of this work. Vada Pinto, M.A. has been a good friend and colleague who, along with the Thursday night group, has taught me much about psychotherapy. Terry Riley, Ph.D. supplied good cigars and conversations on object relations theory. My mother, the Hon. Esther Volkan gave much needed support, while encouraging me to finish this project. My in-laws, Professor Lawrence Kroll, Ph.D. and Kat Kroll deserve thanks for their hospitality during countless San Francisco weekends.

Edward Khantzian, M.D. took time to speak with me and to send a number of his papers. L. Bryce Boyer, M.D. also took time to review the manuscript and to make numerous helpful suggestions. Ellen Spitz, Ph.D. greatly influenced my thinking while I was working on this book and I am grateful for the paper she sent. Margaret Barbee, Ph.D. and Astrid Eiland, Ph.D. have been helpful critics and gave excellent editorial help. I am especially appreciative of the help, criticism, insight, clinical supervision, and friendship I received from Luca DiDonna, Ph.D. It has been a great pleasure to work with such a fine psychologist, music lover, chef and human being. Last, but not least, I would like to thank Leon Wurmser, M.D., who graciously contributed the preface. His paper stands as an erudite piece of scholarship unto itself. I count myself as very fortunate to have the benefit of this fine scholar's perspective and many years of clinical insight.

K.V., Santa Cruz, California

Table of Contents

Preface

By Leon Wurmser, M.D.

"...I kept running up against the fact that our society had made a political choice between two almost equally undesirable outcomes," writes Senator Moynihan in a recent essay in the "American Scholar", quoting Mark Kleiman that,

> in dealing with drugs, we are required to choose between a crime problem and a public health problem. In choosing to prohibit drugs, we choose to have a more or less localized—but ultimately devastating—crime problem rather than a general health problem...This problem now involves 'the structure of authority and governmental legitimacy in America'. ("American Scholar", Vol. 62, No. 3, pp. 355–357)

Thus, substance abuse is a social, legal and political term with strong derogatory, judgmental explicitness, not just connotations.

What has notoriously been given short shrift is the "inner dimension", the personality of the individual drug user, the complex dynamics working behind the facade of the noisy behavioral problems. It is this complexity, i.e., the many layers of theoretical understanding of the mind, which forms the substance of this valuable, well-written, and theoretically as well as clinically instructive and helpful book by Dr. Kevin Volkan. His is a careful and thorough study of the many psychoanalytic and psychoanalytically-informed approaches to the problems of substance abuse. In his rich, panoramic review, Dr.

Volkan uses all the available and commonly accessible perspectives of psychodynamic understanding to answer this double question and to pose new and specific tasks for future research.

He pays particular attention to the new approaches in object relations theory, but sees them as complementary to the more traditional views of intrapsychic conflict—a complementarity which is instructively illuminated by a number of rich case studies, studies not of patients seen by himself, but of several prominent figures from history, literature and mythology, as well as in case studies from the psychoanalytic literature. Central to them is both the exploration of inner conflict as well as of deficiency in interpersonal interaction. He weaves a fascinating tapestry out of the literary and clinical references.

In the remainder of this foreword I would like to add a few considerations of my own that either fill in some of the background to the topic or reflect more recent experiences of mine; both may illustrate the convergence of Dr. Volkan's work and of mine. They deal with the issues of compulsiveness, the causality specific for psychoanalytic explanation, and some observations about technical issues with such severely ill patients, especially the issue of analyzing instead of using the superego transference. (Paul Gray)

What is substance abuse, and what place does compulsive drug use take within that broader frame?

Some authors define substance abuse as any use of a substance affecting the mind for reasons that are not medically accepted and go against the prevailing social and legal standards (Jaffe 1965).

In contrast to this definition based on conformity to some external standards and rules of behavior, it is more consistent with medical tradition, logically and practically, to define substance abuse proper as *the use of any mind-altering substance for the purpose of inner change if it leads to any transient or long range interference with social, cognitive or motor functioning or with physical health,* regardless of the legal and social standing of the substance. It puts the focus on the person and the act instead of arbitrary societal standards. Why should, for example, the drunkenness of a physician at a party not be substance abuse, whereas the often ineffective smoking of one marijuana cigarette would be? Or why should compulsive smoking be any less a form of drug abuse than heroin addiction? Rather, the criterion is here one of the impairment of functioning and health, hence of the definition of psychological normality and illness, transcending its conformity with and adaptation to outer rules.

The clinically most useful classification is that used by the Second Report of the National Commission Marijuana and Drug Abuse (1972), distinguishing five groups: *Experimental use* is a self-limited trial of drugs, primarily motivated by curiosity or the desire to experience new feeling or mood states. *Social or recreational use* occurs in social settings among friends or acquaintances who desire to share an experience perceived by them as both acceptable and pleasurable, usually on a more frequent basis than experimental use. *Circumstantial-situational use* is task-specific and is motivated by the wish to cope with a specific, sometimes recurrent situation or condition of a personal or vocational nature. *Intensified use* is defined as the regular, long-term, patterned use of drugs at a minimum level of at least once daily while still being compatible with social and economic integration and apparent compensation. *Compulsive use* is patterned at both high frequency and high intensity levels of relatively long duration, producing physiological or psychological dependence such that the individual cannot at will discontinue such use without experiencing physiological discomfort or psychological disruption. It is characterized primarily by significantly reduced individual and social functioning.

Using this classification we realize that for practical purposes the first two groups (experimental and social users) appear not to be particularly associated with serious pre-existing psychopathology, whereas the latter two most definitely are, and very many of the third class (situational) as well. We deal here with a continuum, a curve of compulsiveness steeply inclining between classes two and four. This is then rightly the focus of Dr. Volkan's study.

Compulsiveness itself belongs to the very essence of the neurotic process. As Kubie (1954) stressed, the stamp of the *neurotic process is its compulsiveness—its insatiability, automaticity and endless repetitiveness*. To this we may add that the second criterion for the neurotic process consists in the *polarization of the opposites*, the dichotomizing of the judgments of good and bad, of pure and impure, of sacred and demonic, or God and Devil, the extreme quality of love and hate, of trust and distrust. Closely connected with that is the third criterion: the experience of *absoluteness and globality* of most experiences, the claim of totality for affective or cognitive comprehension of self and world. Wishes and affects have a particularly overwhelming, global all-encompassing nature; they cannot be contained. Put in different words: there is an *overvaluation*, an overestimation of self or others; it is a transgressing of the limits, a dissolution of the boundaries, in value, truth and action.

These three then are criteria for *describing* the neurotic process as it becomes glaringly obvious in the severely regressive patients—typically the patients with problems of compulsive substance abuse.

This raises the broader question: What is an addictive behavior? It is evident that many of the current views are urgently in need of revision. There is no such thing as "alcoholism is a disease" in the meaning of a unitary entity with clear and singular cause course and treatment (Fingarette 1988). There is no such thing as an addictive personality with clear and common dynamics and one preferable treatment approach for all. There is no linear relation between one set of causal factors and the symptoms of addictive behavior. There is no sharp line between specific addictions and addictive behavior in general, except for the contingencies of the physical aspects induced by specific drugs; but there is also no sharp line between addictive behavior and the neurotic process. The experiences with the treatment of the severe forms of neurosis, those that now often are singled out either as "narcissistic" or "borderline disorders", are not *principally* separated by a gulf from those with the milder forms, and the problems in the treatment of drug and alcohol dependent patients for the largest part are simply a special form of these severe neuroses.

Addictus is a legal term referring to somebody being given over surrendered, awarded; "addicere liberus corpus in servitutem" means to sentence somebody who is free to servitude because of indebtedness, "addictus" is one in bondage because of debts.

Therefore, metaphorically, addictive behavior refers to a deep *enslaving* dependency on some "thing", some authority, some compelling, constraining force, usually seen and experienced as coming from the outside—a drug, a love partner, food, money, power, gambling—in short, any system or object demanding and getting total submission. It is a seemingly willing subservience to compulsion. In fact, all our psychoanalytic experience tells us that it is neither so "willing" nor that the power is truly on the outside.

For us the problem is: What is this compelling force from *within* that creates such enormously *destructive bondage to something on the outside*? And the one correlated to it: How can we modify or perhaps remove this compulsion?

There is a hidden structure of causality that is specifically relevant to psychoanalytic exploration; it shows the following layers:

1. The psychoanalytic path from description to explanation proceeds from the *core phenomena* of the neurotic process; compulsiveness, polarization and absoluteness—as they typically are reflected in preconscious conflicts, affects and self-protective behaviors.

2. It uses, with particular benefit, the bridges of the *core fantasies* in order to reach,

3. the *unconscious core conflicts.* The recognition of them and the new attempt to resolve them brings about the effective change their place in the inner chain of causal connection is at the very center.

4. Beyond the conflicts we deal with *core affects* of a traumatic or physiologic origin, often determining the severity of the conflicts we deal with. The core fantasies and core conflicts are specifically set up to deal with, to defend against, *central affects of a primary and global nature.*

5. Behind those four layers of psychopathology described, *e.g. phenomena, core fantasies, central conflicts, and main affects*—there looms like a monster, in every case of severe neurosis, the fatal power of *trauma.*

There are of course many forms of traumatization, but of special importance is that what we can call "soul blindness" and "soul murder". "*Soul blindness*" is a systematic, chronic disregard for the emotional needs and expressions of the child, a peculiar blindness to its individuality and hostility to its autonomy. It shows itself as the peculiar dehumanization of the other person, as that what Francis Broucek (1991) has called "objectification" and postulated as the core of the shame experience. As to "*soul murder*", Shengold (1989) defines it as "the deliberate attempt to eradicate or compromise the separate identity of another person...depriving the victim of the ability to feel joy and love as a separate person" (p. 2). It stands "for a certain category of traumatic experience: instances of repetitive and chronic overstimulation, alternating with emotional deprivation, that are deliberately brought about by another individual" (p. 16). It is evident that the first term is subsumed under the second.

In reverse order: The more severe the traumata, the more overwhelming the affects. The more radical and overwhelming the affects, the more intense the conflicts. The more intense and extreme the conflicts, the more encompassing (global) the defenses and the more totalitarian the contradictory demands of "the inner judge", that sadistic version of conscience. Thus the trauma lives on the severity and pitiless character of the conscience as well as in its split character. The more extreme the aggression of the superego, the more life determining are the fantasies and the more prominent the core phenomena described, meaning; the broader the problems of "narcissism", of "splitting of identity", and of compulsiveness.

The use of drugs is part of complex compromise formations and functions in that way as self-therapy. Specifically the drugs block overwhelming affects. They serve in the creation of double reality by aiding the denial both of the traumatic aspects of reality, and more importantly, of the totalitarian aspects of conscience and ideals. They fulfill in complex ways some of the core fantasies of all levels of gratification, and they serve self-punishment.

This view of the *centrality of conflict causality* and the special role in it of conflicts with and within the superego corresponds to a shift in therapeutic emphasis:

First of all, it is crucial not to be beguiled by the manifest drama of drug addiction. Just as it is true for the spectacular phenomenology of multiple personalities or of the perversions, one has to keep in mind that these dramatically displayed phenomena are complex defensive strategies against those underlying fantasies, conflicts, affects and traumata. The *outer compulsion* hides and distracts from the real problem, the *inner compulsion*. The rebellion on the outside is a cover for the inner unfreedom.

Second, in the treatment of patients with "addictive behavior" in particular, with "severe neuroses" in general, special care has to be given not to assume much of a *real* superego role, especially not to be maneuvered into the dilemma between permissiveness and punitiveness, between collusion and prohibition, but rather, as far as this is possible, to analyze the externalized or projected superego functions, as they are manifested in the transference; instead of *using the superego transference*, it should be analyzed—especially in its more subtle forms. It entails avoiding judgmentalness, the exertion of authority, as far as possible, explicitly or implicitly. Yet, when we listen to the case material, such superego *use* cannot always be avoided. Even here there exists a complementarity.

Third, what has been particularly valuable for me is the recommendation that unconscious aggressive or sexual impulses are not treated primarily by confrontation nor direct drive interpretations, but by defense and superego analysis—the *fear* of them rather than their form as wish. The focus is on the many layers of *conflicts* and on the specific range of *affects* they lead to. The traumata, which are refracted by those conflicts, are accessible only through such conflicts.

Fourth, *superego transference means to a large measure sado-masochistic transference.* The analysis of the enormously important role masochism plays in these patients dictates special attention to the problems of trauma and double reality, double consciousness and split identity—as part of the superego pathology.

Fifth, there is no assumption of a superego *defect*, a superego lacuna, but of severe conflicts *within the superego*, nor is there an a priori assumption of visible, deep ego-defects, except for the intolerance towards certain, specific affects; only at the end of thorough conflict analysis is it possible to pinpoint possible ego defects. *Deficit psychology and conflict psychology are two different visions of man;* they are complementary to each other, not an either-or, but they met very different goals and dictate quite different approaches.

Sixth, much importance is given to a rational alliance and hence to a therapeutic atmosphere of kindness and tact, which facilitates such an alliance. In most cases, auxiliary measures—medication, marital or family therapy, self-help groups, even behavioral treatment—are needed because of the severity of affect intolerance and flooding, and hence the severity of conflict and superego pressure; Almost without exception a treatment strategy combining several modalities simultaneously is needed. In that, creativity as part of the treatment is an extremely helpful counterpoise to the destructive compulsion to repeat those masochistic patterns and counterweight to the lasting terror of severe trauma and hitherto unsolvable conflict.

In Dostoyevsky's *Brothers Karamazov*, Lise Khokhlakova asks Alyosha, after he had given her a wonderful "analysis" of the motives for the puzzling and contradictory behavior of the alcoholic and socially, economically and psychologically devastated "Stabskapitan" Snegiryov:

> ...isn't there some contempt for him, for this wretched man...that we're analyzing (razbirayem) his soul like this, as if we were looking down on him?" Alyosha firmly denies this, saying: "...what contempt can there be if we ourselves are just the same as he is, if everyone is just the same as he is? Because we are just the same, not better. And even if we were better, we would still be the same in his place...(trl. Pevear and Volokhonsky, slightly modified by me, p. 217).

The danger of shaming the patient is countered by this fundamental knowledge: much of what the patient suffers and does he shares with us. It may be a mere issue of quantity and circumstance. Ibsen says, in *The Pillars of Society*: "Look into whomever you want, you will in every one at least *one* dark spot he would like to cover" ("Se inn i hvilken mann du vil, og du skal finne i hver eneste en *ett* mørkt punkt i det minste, som han må dekke over"). A similar point is made in the Talmud-tractate Yoma: "One should not appoint anybody to be a leader in the community (parnass al hazibbur), unless he carries on his back a basket full of reptiles (quppa shel shratzim). If he becomes arrogant, one can tell him: Turn around!" (Yoma 22b).

We can be very grateful to Dr. Volkan for this sensitive and non-judgmental, rich and helpful compendium. In its multiplicity of perspectives and forms of understanding, but also in its avoiding that danger of judgmentalness, it evokes in me the message reflected in the following story in the Talmud:

There was a bitter dispute between Rabbi Yochanan and his former pupil Resh Laqish, in which they deeply humiliated each other. Resh Laqish fell ill and his wife pleaded with Rabbi Yochanan, her brother, to forgive her husband the slight. He refused, and Resh Laqish died. Now Rabbi Yochanan was overtaken by remorse and grief.

> Said the Rabbis: 'Who shall go to ease his mind? Let R. Eleazar ben Pedath go, whose disquisitions are very subtle.' So he went and sat before him; and on every dictum uttered by R. Yochanan he observed: 'There is a Baraitha (a taught opinion) which supports you.' 'Are you as the son of Laqisha?' he complained: 'When I stated a law, the son of Laqisha used to raise twenty-four objections, to which I gave twenty-four answers, which consequently led to a fuller comprehension of the law; whilst you say: "A Baraitha has been taught which supports you." Do I not myself know that my dicta are right?' Thus he went on rending his garments and weeping: 'Where are you, o son of Laqisha, where are you, o son of Laqisha! ("hecha at Bar Laqisha, hecha at Bar Laqisha!")' and he cried thus until his mind was turned. Thereupon the Rabbis prayed for him, and he died" (Bava Metzia, 84a; H. Freedman, ed. I Epstein).

L.W., Towson, Maryland
August 8, 1993

Chapter One

Introduction

At 3:30 in the afternoon, August 16, 1977, Elvis Aaron Presley was pronounced dead at the Baptist Memorial Hospital in Memphis Tennessee. The cause of death was officially listed as cardiac arrhythmia. Those who were close to Elvis, however, suspected a different cause: compulsive drug use. Although strongly opposed to illegal drugs, Elvis had been a compulsive user of powerful medications prescribed by various physicians. For many years he had used stimulants, depressants and steroids on a regular basis. This drug use eventually took a heavy toll on the body and mind of Elvis Presley.

Just as Elvis' heart failure can be attributed to his history of drug use, his drug use can be attributed to an underlying psychopathological condition. Indeed, on close examination one notices many irregularities in Elvis' personal history such as, being a surviving twin, his father's absence during his infancy, sleeping with his parents until his teens, the need to maintain a familiar and controlled environment, rapid mood swings, poor psychological boundaries, etc. Of course, it is impossible to know the complete details of Elvis' childhood, including his and his parents' unconscious fantasies. For instance, it is impossible to know what Elvis' parents experienced having one twin die and the other live during childbirth, or what the impact was of Elvis' loss of his father during his early childhood. Although nothing definitive

can be said about Elvis' internal intrapsychic world, these irregularities in Elvis' history can be suspected of having a relationship to the development of his drug habit and indeed,
are common themes in the lives of many compulsive drug
users. Nevertheless, it is not generally known how these
psychological irregularities interact to create a compulsive
drug habit. Psychologists have searched for the crucial in-
gredient that causes one person to become a drug addict and
another to perhaps try drugs and then lose interest. As Elvis'
death indicates, compulsive drug use often has tragic consequences.

   While biological and genetic factors are undoubtedly important in understanding drug use, they have of late, been
overemphasized. It is my contention that much of our understanding of drug use is seriously flawed and at odds with
psychoanalytic theories of psychopathology.

   For instance, Shedler and Block (1990) have recently produced research findings which seriously question the prevailing notions of drug use. These researchers investigated
the relationship between drug use and a number of psychological characteristics among adolescents who were tracked
longitudinally from early childhood to age eighteen. They
found that adolescents who had some experience with drugs
were the most well-adjusted. Those adolescents who had
never used drugs were found to be anxious, emotionally
constricted and lacking social skills. Finally, those adolescents who used drugs frequently were found to suffer from a
distinct personality syndrome characterized by interpersonal
alienation, impulsiveness and emotional distress. Shedler
and Block concluded that the psychological characteristics of
these three groups of adolescents (occasional users, abstain-
ers and frequent users) were due to the quality of parenting
they had received. They also concluded that frequent drug
use is a symptom of a deeper pathology due to early childhood trauma and therefore, many drug prevention efforts
are misguided because they focus upon the symptoms of
drug use rather than addressing early psychological problems.

   Since the Shedler and Block study, mental health workers, educators and public health officials now face a peculiar

dilemma. They are in the unenviable position of having to respond to the posturing of public officials and a media blitz which, is not only lacking in scientific credibility, but is also of questionable efficacy. This contradiction has led many professionals to become confused about drug use, its treatment, and prevention. Yet, many in the psychological community have been vindicated by the Shedler and Block study. This is especially true for psychoanalytic psychotherapists and psychoanalysts who have held a viewpoint similar to Shedler and Block's since the time of Freud. Given the high cost to society of drug use, it is my opinion that the understanding of the psychology of the drug user is an underlying key issue and should get treatment at least equal to legal, social and political issues.

Freud and Drugs

Freud was the first psychologist to study and experience what we would now label a dangerous drug. This drug was cocaine. Starting in 1884 and extending through 1887, Freud studied the effects of cocaine. His hope was that the discovery of medical uses for the drug would catapult him into fame and allow him to marry his fiancé earlier than had been planned. In fact, it was Freud who first suggested that the anesthetic properties of cocaine might be useful for eye surgery, although it was Freud's contemporary Carl Koller who successfully demonstrated this use of the drug. Freud's friend and mentor, Wilhelm Fliess repeatedly prescribed cocaine for Freud, who became a regular user. Freud wrote,

> If it goes well I will write an essay on it and I expect it will win its place in therapeutics, by the side of morphia and superior to it. I have other hopes and intentions about it. I take very small doses of it regularly against depression and against indigestion, and with the most brilliant success…in short it is only now that I feel I am a doctor. (Jones, 1961, p. 54)

Freud soon became an evangelist for cocaine use and in the words of Jones (1961), he "…was rapidly becoming a public menace" (p. 55).

It was only after he had advised his friend Ernst von Fleischl-Marxow to use cocaine that Freud's enthusiasm for the drug began to pale. Von Fleischl-Marxow had accidentally contracted a severe infection in his hand during a laboratory experiment. The accident required the amputation of von Fleischl-Marxow's thumb to save his life. Yet he was never quite cured, as the residual infection caused recurrent tumors which had to be removed. Von Fleischl-Marxow had become a morphine addict in his quest to find relief from the continual and severe pain he experienced. Freud suggested that von Fleischl-Marxow try cocaine in order to relieve his pain and to wean him from morphine. At first, it seemed as if the cocaine was successful. It alleviated von Fleischl-Marxow's morphine addiction and provided some relief. This relief, however, was short-lived as von Fleischl-Marxow required increasingly larger doses, until he was taking hundreds of times a normal dose. Freud watched as cocaine destroyed his friend with the realization that it was not the panacea he had envisioned. Freud, at first, blamed von Fleischl-Marxow's problem on the fact that the cocaine was injected with a hypodermic needle, but as reports of cocaine dependence increased he could no longer hide from the truth (Jones, 1961). He later wrote,

> I had been the first to recommend the use of cocaine, in 1884, and this recommendation had brought serious reproaches down on me. The misuse of that drug had hastened the death of a dear friend of mine. (Freud, 1900, p. 144)

Freud puzzled over why cocaine, which was seemingly harmless to himself, was destructively addicting to others. He concluded that there must be present in the personality of the addict, some pathological element, of which he was free[1] (Jones, 1961).

Freud's psychoanalytic method has made great strides towards identifying this element of pathology. This book is a

---

[1] Of course we know that Freud was severely addicted to tobacco and therefore, was not free of addictive pathology. In fact, Freud suffered greatly from ill-health caused by smoking tobacco and eventually died as a result of it.

further attempt to understand the psychopathology of drug use within the context of the psychoanalytic method. Beginning with Chapter Two, I will discuss ways of conceptualizing drug use and the different types of drugs and their effects. Also discussed in this chapter is the research literature on the external (non-psychodynamic) factors related to drug use. Starting with Chapter Three, I will begin to examine the inner world of the drug user. This chapter will outline the varying psychoanalytic descriptions of compulsive drug use. In Chapter Four I will continue to describe the inner world of the compulsive drug user, this time from the standpoint of object relations theory. Chapter Five will outline the support for the use of case studies from clinical settings, the published literature, and historical and mythological figures in psychoanalytic research and present case material which is descriptive of the points made in the previous chapters. Finally, in Chapter Six I will further detail the implications of a psychoanalytic theory of compulsive drug for clinical practice and social policy.

Chapter Two

Varieties of Drug Use Pathology

Drug use as a psychopathological disorder occupies a gray area. Different cultures and societies take differing views of the use of psychoactive substances. For example, use of peyote by Native Americans is an integral part of their religion. Beetlenut, a mild stimulant, is used with impunity in India and many parts of Asia. The use of alcohol made from fermented fruits or grains is practically a universal feature of human culture. Coffee, tea, nicotine and a host of other substances are used regularly by a large percentage of the world's population. Some writers have even claimed that drug use is the result of a naturally occurring human drive to alter one's consciousness (Weil & Rosen, 1983)[1]. What, then, makes drug use pathological? For the most part the answer can be divided into three categories; Environmental and Societal Prohibition, Political Prohibition, and Maladaptive Behavior Change.

Under the category of Environmental and Social Prohibition, drug use is considered pathological because it goes against established beliefs and rules of society. These rules, in some cases, were established because the resultant

---

[1] More comprehensive psychologies such as psychoanalysis, do not, of course, believe in such a drive. The apparent observation of a human drive to alter one's consciousness may be due to the widespread use of mind-altering substances in human cultures. Nevertheless, it is my belief that drug use is not due to an underlying conscious-altering drive, but to the nature of human development, which has universal features.

behaviors or attitudes of drug use pose a threat to the environmental safety of a society. In other cases, the rules and prohibitions seem arbitrary and are not apparently related to the establishment of a safe environment. An example of the former case would be the prohibition of alcohol use by oil tanker captains while on duty. As demonstrated by the wreck of the *Exxon Valdez* in Alaska, drug use can have serious environmental consequences for our society. An example of the latter case would be the prohibition of coffee drinking by members of the Mormon religion. While no doubt having significance within this group, the negative impact to society at large is less clear.

The second category of apparently psychopathological drug use would be primarily political in nature. Although it is rarely mentioned, some psychoactive substances cause the user to question his society, values, culture and self. Therefore, individuals and institutions which have a vested interest in maintaining the *status quo* find it convenient to label the use of certain drugs by certain people as pathological. A well-documented example of this is the suppression of the use of LSD in the United States. The book *Acid Dreams* by Lee and Shlain (1985) tells the story of how LSD was studied by the CIA as a psychomimetic agent for mind control. During the course of this experiment, LSD was introduced into the general population and became a cornerstone for the counter-culture of the 60's. The effects of the drug soon set the tenor and climate for the 60's, a time of youthful rebellion and uninhibited expression. Although LSD can have seriously harmful effects (Seymor & Smith, 1987), especially among those with a predilection towards mental illness, it is physically one of the least harmful psychoactive substances known. In the 1950's LSD research was a legitimate line of inquiry and the 'good' effects of the drug were studies in controlled clinical settings. By and large this research involved giving LSD to alcoholic and obsessive patients to see if it would increase levels of insight and 'loosen them up'. In the space of a few years, however, LSD became a 'bad' drug and most of the research on its effects in therapy was halted. Much scientific information about LSD has been severely suppressed and misinformation has been disseminated with such efficiency, that it is commonly thought to be an extremely dangerous drug. However, a review of the published research on LSD shows good effects, especially when it is used under supervision in a clinical setting (Grof, 1973, Ling & Buckman, 1965). The slander campaign against LSD has even been successful in eliminating most scientific research into the medical uses of LSD. Other drugs have also had the same treatment as LSD, the most notable recent example being MMDA and MDMA, the so-called 'designer drugs'. These drugs, although possibly more physically harmful than LSD, also produce heightened awareness and sensitivity and hence, are thought to be useful in conjunction with psychotherapy (Rosenbaum & Doblin, 1990). While it is certainly not the purpose here to argue the politics of drug use, it is clear that the label of psychopathology can work as a political tool. Nevertheless, most psychotherapists would undoubtedly question the place of such politicization of psychopathology in a truly free society. Although the political ramifications of drug use would make an interesting topic for study, they will not be elaborated on here (cf. Szasz, 1992).

The third definition of psychopathological drug use is that of maladaptive mood and behavior change. This definition represents the most common psychological understanding of the psychopathology of drug use, although it often overlaps with the first definition. As noted earlier, change in mood and behavior would be considered positive in some societies and negative in another. In other words, the psychopathology of drug use represented here can be understood to cause individual suffering in both the short- and long-term. According to the *Diagnostic and Statistical Manual of Mental Disorders, Third Edition Revised* (DSM III-R) of the American Psychiatric Association (1987) drug use psychopathology consists of symptoms and maladaptive behavioral changes associated with habitual use of a drug that affects the central nervous system. These symptoms and behavior changes need to be understood as universally maladaptive among all human cultures. Although it would be difficult to agree on a universal definition of what type of drug use is maladaptive, the DSM III-R lists such criteria as continued use of a drug despite the intractability of social, occupational, psychological, or physical problems that are clearly exacerbated by drug use, and the development of withdrawal symptoms. The DSM III-R goes on to state,

> The conditions are here conceptualized as mental disorders, and are therefore to be distinguished from non-pathological psychoactive substance use, such as moderate imbibing of alcohol or the use of certain substances for appropriate medical purposes. (p. 165)

The pathological patterns under this definition can be broken into the categories of *substance dependence* and *substance abuse*. While these two categories are useful for conceptualizing drug use, there is often a significant overlap between the two. Recent research, although controversial, has indicated that drug use follows a progression starting with milder or 'soft' drugs, like marijuana or tobacco, and ends up with dependence or addiction to dangerous or 'hard' drugs, like heroin or crack cocaine (Kandel, Kessler & Margulies, 1978). The ultimate stage of drug use pathology is usually understood as addiction to opiates. This addiction often takes place after a prolonged history of polydrug abuse (Blatt, Rounsaville, Eyre & Wilber, 1984).

There is some confusion about the terminology used to describe different levels and types of drug use pathology. Both categories of *dependence* and *abuse* will be used here, with *substance dependence* signifying greater pathology than *substance abuse*. The term *compulsive drug use* is also used to indicate substance abuse with addictive qualities, regardless of the type of drug. The terms *drug* and *substance* will be used equivalently. The term drug or substance *use* will represent use of drugs without specifying the level of pathology (abuse or dependence).

In general, substance dependence is marked by a greater frequency and variety of symptoms than substance abuse. The DSM III-R (1987, p. 167-168) lists the diagnostic criteria for substance dependence, which are paraphrased below;

1. The substance is often taken in larger amounts or over a longer period of time than the person intended;

2. There is a persistent desire or one or more unsuccessful efforts to cut down or control substance use;

3. A great deal of time is spent in activities necessary to get the substance (e.g. theft), taking the substance (e.g. chain smoking), or recovering from its effects;

4. There is frequent intoxication or withdrawal symptoms when the person is expected to fulfill major role obligations at work, school, or home (e.g. does not go to work because hung over, goes to school or work "high", intoxicated while taking care of his or her children), or when substance use is physically hazardous (e.g. drives when intoxicated);

5. Important social, occupational, or recreational activities are given up or reduced because of substance use;

6. There is continued substance use despite knowledge of having a persistent or recurrent social, psychological, or physical problem that is caused or exacerbated by the use of the substance (e.g. keeps using heroin despite family arguments about it, cocaine-induced depression, or having an ulcer made worse by drinking);

7. A marked tolerance or need for markedly increased amounts of the substance (i.e., at least a 50% increase) in order to achieve intoxication or desired effect with continued use of the same amount;

8. Characteristic withdrawal symptoms;

9. The substance is often taken to relieve or avoid withdrawal symptoms.

The presence of at least three of the above criteria, along with evidence that some symptoms of the disturbance have persisted for at least one month, or have occurred repeatedly over a longer period of time, are necessary for the diagnosis of substance dependence.

Substance abuse is a category in the DSM III-R (1987) for recording maladaptive behavior patterns which do not meet the diagnostic criteria for substance dependence. The criteria for substance abuse, paraphrased from the DSM III-R (1987, p. 169) are as follows;

1. Continued use of a substance despite knowledge of having a persistent or recurrent social, occupational, psychological, or physical problem that is caused or exacerbated by the use of the psychoactive substance.

2. Recurrent use of the substance in situations in which use is physically hazardous (e. g. driving while intoxicated).

A diagnosis of substance abuse requires at least one of the above criteria. In addition, this diagnosis requires that the symptoms of the disturbance have persisted for at least one month, or have occurred repeatedly over a longer period of time and that the person has never met the criteria for substance dependence.

The DSM III-R (1987) also lists nine classes of psychoactive substances. Each of these (with exception of nicotine, which is generally considered a problem of substance dependence) is associated with both abuse and dependence. The substances are alcohol, amphetamine or similar substance, cannabis, cocaine, hallucinogens, inhalants, opiates, phencyclidine (PCP) or similar substance, and sedatives, hypnotics, or anxiolytics. A brief description for each substance taken from the DSM III-R and other sources (Levin, 1987; Seymor & Smith, 1987) is listed below.

Alcohol

Alcohol, ethanol, or ethyl alcohol is produced through the fermentation of sugars by yeast. This drug has been present in some form throughout human history. It is still the most widely used and abused drug of choice in the United States.

People vary widely in their tolerance to alcohol. Some of this tolerance is the result of genetic variation in the enzymatic ability to process alcohol in the body. Tolerance to alcohol also increases with use. Alcohol consumption typically follows one of three patterns. The first pattern is daily intake of large quantities, the second is regular weekend bingeing, and the third is long periods of sobriety punctuated with daily binges of heavy drinking which persist for weeks or months. The onset of alcoholism typically occurs during the late teens and early 20's for males. The disease is more variable with females. For example, their onset is usually later and also often associated with mood disorders, although dependence upon alcohol is commonly associated with depression in both sexes. Alcohol is often used with other drugs and this associated polydrug abuse is most often found among teenagers. Middle-aged people commonly use alcohol with tranquilizers (benzodiazepines). Nicotine dependence is common among alcohol abusers of all ages. It has also been shown that alcohol dependence can be transmitted from generation to generation without the presence of the dependent family members. Alcohol dependency, however, has been shown to have a genetic component.

The effect of alcohol is to depress the central nervous system. At small doses, alcohol releases inhibitions and produces minor behavior changes and a general elevation of mood. At higher doses, marked behavior change takes place. This behavior can become increasingly violent and paranoid. At massive doses, the central nervous system can be profoundly depressed, resulting in death.

Amphetamines and Related Substances

This class of drugs includes methamphetamine, dextroamphetamine, amphetamine, and various 'designer drugs' such as MMDA, which are chemically similar to amphetamine. These drugs are stimulants which are taken orally, intravenously or nasally. A form of the drug called 'ice', which can be smoked, has also recently become prevalent. This class of drugs was once widely prescribed for weight loss, but is now reserved for those with severe weight problems or narcolepsy. People self-prescribe amphetamines for a variety of reasons which do not fall under the legal uses of the drug. Truck drivers and students commonly take amphetamines to stay awake and maintain concentration for long periods of time. Physicians and combat pilots have also been known to take amphetamines for this reason. Amphetamine use usually falls into one of three patterns, episodic use, chronic daily use, or almost daily use. Bingeing is common with users taking high doses for short periods of time followed by a few days of recuperation. The binges tend to end when the supply of the drug and/or the users become exhausted. The period of recuperation is referred to a "crash". During this time the user experiences profound depression as well as physical depletion. Users of ice no doubt have a worse crash experience because smoking the drug leads to a higher concentration of the drug in the body in a shorter amount of time. Amphetamine abusers will often take other drugs, usually alcohol or a narcotic. The amphetamine user typically demonstrates impulsively and rapid mood changes. At high doses, toxic psychosis can occur, mimicking a paranoid delusional state. Withdrawal from the drug has been associated with depression, general irritability, anergia and isolation. Intravenous users tend to progress to dependence faster than those who use the drug nasally or orally. Tolerance to amphetamines takes place rapidly.

Cannabis

Cannabis derives its psychoactive properties from tetrahydrocannabinol (THC) which is present in the leaves and flowers of the plant. The plant is usually smoked but can be eaten to give a longer lasting effect. Cannabis has some documented medical uses such as relief of eye pressure in glaucoma and the relief of nausea in patients undergoing chemotherapy treatment for cancer. Cannabis use is common and it is probably the most widely used illegal drug in America. Although many people use Cannabis, the rate of abuse and dependence on this drug is fairly low (McVay, 1991; Smith, 1970). The acceptance of Cannabis in America is such that many communities have substantially reduced the penalties for possession of the drug, resulting in *defacto* legalization (McVay, 1991). Cannabis dependence and abuse usually develops over a long period of time. The user does not generally develop a tolerance to the drug and in fact may need smaller doses after repeated use. Generally, it is the frequency of use rather than the amount used that increases over time. Cannabis dependence and abuse is related to maladaptive behavior, short term memory impairment and dysphoria.

Cocaine

Cocaine is derived from the leaves of the coca plant which is indigenous to South America. In its native countries, coca leaves are chewed for their mild stimulant effect. Aside from some dental problems, chewing coca leaves does not appear to be a harmful practice. Cocaine is removed from the coca leaves through chemical processes which result in the production of cocaine hydrochloride powder. This powder is usually taken nasally or through intravenous injection. Recently, the cocaine alkaloid has been purified from the powder into a smokeable form of the drug commonly called "crack". The crack form of cocaine is smoked and the effects of the drug are experienced very rapidly. Cocaine use is similar to the use of amphetamines with episodic use, chronic daily use and almost daily use. Bingeing is also common and is commonly associated with crack smoking. The crash at the end of a binge is also similar to experience of the amphetamine user, though the crash for the crack smoker (like the ice user) appears to be dramatically worse. This may be due to profound changes in neurotransmitter levels in the brain of the crack user. The behavioral and mood changes, and the course of use associated with cocaine use are similar to those caused by amphetamine use.

Hallucinogens

This category includes man-made drugs related to LSD, DMT, MDA, and organically occurring substances like mescaline and psilocybin. Most hallucinogens are taken orally, although other modalities of administration are sometimes used. Patterns of use are highly variable. Evidence indicates that most users experiment only a few times with these drugs. Anecdotal evidence suggests that for most people there are three stages of hallucinogen use. The first stage is an experimental one in which a user finds out whether or not he likes the drug. If the user finds the drug enjoyable he may begin to take it on an episodic regular basis. After a period of time, which depends on the amount of the drug taken and the frequency of use, the user will begin to become bored or disillusioned with the psychedelic experience. Many users at this point will say that there is nothing more for the drug to "teach" them and they will stop using the drug abruptly. Although the literature indicates that users build a tolerance to hallucinogens, the quality of these drugs is so variable that this is virtually impossible to determine. Dependence on hallucinogens is very rare and most users return to a normal pattern of life after a short period of use.

Inhalants

These drugs are usually made up of hydrocarbons such as found in glue, hair-spray, paint, paint thinner, typewriter correction fluid, spray paint and even gasoline. Little is known about the different effects of these substances except that they are all capable of producing some type of "high". As the name implies, these substances are administered by breathing in their fumes through the nose and mouth. Inhalant users have been found to originate from highly dysfunctional families and have a number of other complicating problems including use of other drugs, delinquency, truancy, etc. There are higher incidences of inhalant use among the lower socioeconomic classes. Inhalant users generally start at a young age, typically with a peer group who are abusing alcohol and cannabis. Inhalant use can increase until it becomes the drug of choice for the user. Dependence on inhalants has been documented for industrial workers who have been exposed to these substances in the workplace over long periods of time. These workers may begin using the inhalant for its psychoactive effect. Inhalant users experience many medical complications including kidney and liver disease. These problems can arise from even occasional use.

Nicotine

Nicotine, derived from the tobacco plant, is a naturally occurring pesticide and is one of the most addictive drugs known to man. The DSM III-R (1987) does not list nicotine abuse as a category because it is assumed that all users will become dependent on the drug. The most common form of nicotine use is cigarette smoking. Other forms of use include cigar and pipe smoking as well as chewing tobacco and snuff. These less common forms of tobacco use are relatively less likely to lead to dependence and medical problems. Nicotine causes and aggravates a number of serious medical complaints. Anxiety over the possible medical problems caused by the drug are reported by many users. In recent years there has been increasing social pressure to quit smoking in the form of workplace prohibitions and city ordinances banning smoking in public places. Nicotine dependence develops rapidly and most users fail at numerous attempts to stop using the drug. Relapse only becomes uncommon after the user has abstained for at least a year.

Opiates

These substances are either man-made or derived from the opium poppy. Many opiates have legitimate medical uses such as analgesics and anesthetics. Opiates are usually taken orally or intravenously, but may also be taken nasally or smoked. Opiate dependence sometimes develops from a legitimate use, such as treatment by a physician for pain. Most often, however, users try the drug in an illegal form in their late teens or early twenties after using many different types of drugs. The use of opiates is often peer oriented and many aspects of the use of the drug are ritualized, including needle sharing which puts opiate addicts at risk for contracting diseases such as HIV. (See D. Rosenfeld, 1992, p. 236 for a discussion of ritual needle sharing). After a user is addicted to an opiate, the procurement and use of the drug comes to dominate their existence. Recovery from opium dependence is related to the context of the drug use. Many of the soldiers who became addicts during the Vietnam War have been able to relinquish the habit once they were back in the United States (Zinberg, 1975). Most addicts, however, become involved in a pattern that is repeated over a long period of time. This pattern includes periods of remission from dependence, usually while in a treatment center or prison. Some addicts, provided they can survive the violence-prone lifestyle associated with procuring the drug, are better able to abstain and kick the habit after an average of nine years. Other addicts continue to be dependent throughout their lives.

Phencyclidine

This group includes Phencyclidine (PCP) and other man-made substances. These drugs can be taken in almost any mode; nasally, orally, intravenously and by smoking. Most users are exposed to PCP when it is mixed with other substances. A user will take a drug (usually cannabis) and notice that its effect is different. The user will subsequently find out that this difference is due to the addition of PCP to their drug. If the user likes the effect he will then seek out PCP specifically. Many users are experimental, finding the effects of the drug to be highly variable. These experimenters discontinue using PCP almost immediately. PCP abuse or dependence develops after a short period of occasional regular use. PCP is usually taken in binges that can last several days, although daily chronic use is also commonly reported. It is not clear whether or not tolerance or withdrawal symptoms develop from PCP use.

Sedatives

This group includes substances ranging from mild tranquilizers to barbiturates. Although these substances are very different, they all produce similar effects. They are commonly prescribed by physicians, and usually taken orally. Patterns of use are similar to opiates. Some users start taking sedatives under a physician's prescription, while other users start taking these drugs with a peer group as teens or young adults. Tolerance develops rapidly as do withdrawal symptoms upon cessation of use of these drugs. Episodic use soon leads to chronic use as a tolerance to the drug develops. Chronic use is strongly related to an increase in drug seeking behavior. Although sedatives are highly addicting, many people stop using these drugs and recover from their dependence. Withdrawal from some sedatives is very dangerous and should be done under a physician's supervision.

Use of Multiple Substances

In addition to the above categories, many people use a number of different drugs without a clear drug of choice. These users are classified as *polysubstance dependent, psychoactive substance dependent not otherwise specified* or, *psychoactive substance abuse not otherwise specified*. The classification category of polysubstance dependence is used when at least three substances (excluding caffeine and nicotine) are used repeatedly for six months or longer. The categories of psychoactive substance abuse and dependence not otherwise specified represent residual categories for substance use that does not fall into one of the other groups.

Prevalence of Drug Use

Drug use in the United States rose dramatically in the 1960's and 70's and then leveled off to a fairly consistent level (Falco, 1988). In 1962 it was estimated that 4% of the population had tried an illegal drug. By 1982 this percentage rose to 33%. The cost to society of substance abuse has been estimated to be between ten- and twenty-billion dollars per year in the United States (Seymor & Smith, 1987). Substance abuse is perhaps most notably prevalent in adolescence, during which time most initiation into drug use takes place (Thorne and Deblassie, 1985). According to Wurmser (1987), "The treatment of compulsive drug use is nearly always related to the issues of adolescence and early adulthood" (p. 157). A recent survey reports that nearly 80% of adolescents have tried an illegal drug and roughly 60% have tried illegal drugs other than, or in addition to marijuana, by the time they are in their mid-20s. Approximately 65% of high school seniors use alcohol on a monthly basis and 37% drink heavily on occasion. Daily cigarette smoking has been reported by 18% of high school students (Johnson, O'Malley & Bachman, 1987).

The health hazards of cigarettes and alcohol are well known. These two substances are leading contributors to mortality through either disease or traumatic accident (Statistical Bulletin, 1984; Surgeon General, 1979; Sutton, 1983). The effects of marijuana use are less clear, but there is evidence of negative physiological and psychological effects from long-term intensive use and impairment of cognitive function in the short term (Haas, 1987; Institute of Medicine, 1982; Peterson, 1984). Other studies, however, have shown that marijuana use can increase feelings of self-acceptance and social cohesion among users (Bentler, 1987; Greaves, 1980).

Drugs such as cocaine and narcotics have been reported to be dangerous (Chasnoff, 1987; Duncan, 1987). These substances are especially addicting and contribute directly and indirectly to the spread of diseases, including HIV infection (Battjes & Pickens, 1988; Chatlos, 1987; Falco, 1988; Ravenholt, 1984). These facts are especially of concern when it is estimated that up to 10% of those who try drugs are at risk for becoming addicted (Seymor & Smith, 1987).

Exogenous Factors Affecting Drug Use

There is an extensive literature on the antecedents of drug use. Much, if not most, of this literature is based on studies of exogenous factors, i.e. social, environmental, interpersonal and behavioral factors. Although it is almost impossible to find a consensus among different research studies about the antecedents of drug use, there is enough overlap to allow the construction of broad categories (Newcomb, Maddhian & Bentler, 1986; Wallack & Corbett, 1987; Perry & Murray, 1985; Hawkins, Lishner & Catalano, 1986). These categories can be conceptualized as *demographic, social-environmental, interpersonal* and *behavioral*.

Among the demographic factors affecting drug use are sex, age, ethnicity, geographic region and socioeconomic status. In general, men are more likely than women to use alcohol and illicit drugs (Ensminger, Brown & Kellam, 1982; Johnston, O'Malley & Bachman, 1987; Kandel & Logan, 1984): minorities appear more likely to use drugs than Caucasians, (although some studies have disagreed with these findings, cf. Keyes & Block, 1984): and non-college bound students are more likely to use drugs than college bound students. Early age of onset of any drug use may be the best predictor of future drug use (Kandel, 1975; Kandel & Faust, 1975; Kandel, Kessler and Margulies, 1978; Hawkins, Lishner and Catalano, 1986). Although these demographic variables are related to substance use, they are not as strongly related as the social, environmental, interpersonal or behavioral factors (Perry & Murray, 1985).

The social and environmental factors related to drug use have been extensively studied in adolescent populations. These studies have focused upon three institutions or groups in society; families, schools and peers. The extent to which adolescents—one of the largest groups of drug users—interact with these groups is particularly important (Ensminger, Brown & Kellam, 1982; Hundleby & Mercer, 1987; Jessor,

1979; Kandel, 1980; Kandel & Adler, 1982; Marcos & Bahr, 1988). Adolescents are more likely to use drugs if their family or peers approve, tolerate or model drug use (Brook, Whiteman, Scovell & Brenden, 1983; Johnson, Shontz & Locke, 1984; Smith, Koob, & Wirtz, 1985). Adolescents are also more likely to use drugs if parent and peer values are in conflict and the adolescent is weakly integrated into the home and strongly bonded with friends who exert pressure to use substances (Babst, Miran, & Koval, 1976; Jessor, Jessor & Finney, 1973; Meeks, 1985; Mijuskovic, 1988). Finally, adolescents are more likely to use drugs if they are loosely bonded with their school (Hawkins, Lishner, Catalano, & Howard, 1986; Hawkins, Jenson, Catalano & Lishner, 1988).

Interpersonal factors associated with drug use include a variety of factors related to failure or nonconformity. The factors are: valuation of independence, valuation of lower achievement, greater expectation of failure (low self-efficacy), low assertiveness, low religiosity, greater tolerance of deviant behavior, greater criticism of authority and social institutions, greater rebelliousness, low social conformity, increased receptivity to new ideas and experiences, increased interest in spontaneity and creativity, and increased stress and negative life change events (Dielhman, Campanelli, Shope & Butchart, 1987; Horan & Williams, 1982; Newcomb & Harlow, 1986; Perry & Murray, 1985; Segal, 1986).

Finally, behavioral factors that may affect drug use include early sexual activity, poor academic performance, the use of other legal or illegal drugs and delinquent behaviors. Several studies have indicated that the use of cigarettes and illegal drugs are interrelated (Coomb, Fawzy & Gerber, 1984; Jessor, Jessor & Finney, 1973; Kandel & Logan, 1984; Yamaguchi & Kandel, 1984a, 1984b). Research has suggested that many of these behaviors precede drug use as well as follow it. Some researchers have shown that it can be constructive to think of the variables in the demographic, social, environmental, interpersonal and behavioral categories as risk factors in an epidemiological model (Newcomb, Maddahian & Bentler, 1986; Bry, McKeon & Pandrina, 1982). These studies have supported the idea the number of risk factors is positively and linearly associated with drug use.

Thus, even though individual factors related to the etiology of substance use have been identified, there is no single exogenous factor that accounts for drug use. In the words of one review,

> This view supports previous reviews of the substance abuse literature which have found a variety of etiological or predisposing factors to substance abuse that elude parsimonious conceptual integration. (Newcomb, Maddhian & Bentler, 1986, p. 529)

In a previous paper (K. Volkan & Fetro, 1990), I have attempted to clarify this confusion by elucidating the psychological and social underpinnings of drug use in order to identify the components necessary for the creation of successful drug use prevention programs. My review suggests that most research on drug use has focused more on exogenous environmental factors than on endogenous internal psychodynamic factors. Notwithstanding the usefulness of the demographic and epidemiological research into the exogenous factors related to drug use, it is my opinion (along with others) that this research is theoretically vacant with regards to the intrapsychic developmental factors leading to the compulsive use of drugs (Wurmser, 1974). More importantly, it could be misleading with regard to the prevention and treatment of pathological drug use (Shedler & Block, 1990). Although exogenous factors obviously play an important role in the explanation of drug use, I believe that this role can not be fully understood until the endogenous factors related to drug use are elucidated.

Chapter Three

Psychoanalytic Theories of Drug Use and Addiction

The area of psychology that has given close study to the endogenous factors which influence and shape the personality is psychoanalytic theory. This body of knowledge is perhaps the best tool to illuminate intrapsychic entities such as unconscious fantasies and mental representations. Included among these entities are fantasies and mental representations of drugs, i.e. what drugs mean to the user above and beyond their physiological effect.

Psychoanalytic theory also describes the course of human development and accounts for deviations in normal development due to psychological conflict and trauma in the growing child. Therefore, psychoanalytic theory is useful for elucidating the early childhood conflicts and deviations from the normal developmental course experienced by compulsive drug users.

Psychoanalytic theory has been extremely useful in understanding compulsive or addictive behaviors other than drug use. Compulsive behaviors such as obligatory sexual deviations and the use of inanimate objects other than drugs which are not taken into the body (i.e. eaten or injected) have been extensively studied in the psychoanalytic literature (Abraham, 1910; Freud, 1927; Greenacre, 1969, 1970; V. Volkan & Kavanaugh, 1988) This research has found that some people have a compulsory need for deriving pleasure from inanimate objects like shoes, clothing, etc. In these fetishes, the visual or tactile properties of an inanimate object is used in a compulsory fashion to reach orgasm. Since psychoanalytic theory has been useful for the study of the compulsory fetishes it stands to be useful for the study of compulsive drug use.

A number of psychoanalytically-oriented studies have also tackled the problem of treating the drug user either through psychoanalysis alone or in combination with other treatment modalities (Abadi, 1984; Brill, 1977; Berthelsdorf, 1976; Clerici, 1986; Edelstein, 1975; DeAngelis, 1975; Fine, 1972; Ghaffari, 1987; Gottesfeld, Caroff & Lieberman, 1972; Grenier, 1985; Khantzian, 1987a, 1987b, 1989; Lidz, Lidz & Rubenstein, 1976; Miller, 1983; Radford, Wiseberg & Yorke, 1971; Wurmser, 1985, 1987). A few such programs have claimed some measured success with at least a partially psychoanalytic approach (Grenier, 1985; Schiffer, 1988). These treatment programs have, by and large, been derived from the psychoanalytic literature into the nature of compulsive drug use.

Classical Psychoanalytic Literature on Compulsive Drug Use

Freud (1928, 1985) conceptualized addictionas being related to the habit of masturbation, with its pleasurable and non-pleasurable aspects. In Freud's conceptualization, drugs are substitutions for masturbation (H. Rosenfeld, 1965). The act of masturbation itself gives instinctual gratification, but is forbidden by parental authority which the individual assimilates into his own psychic system (superego system). The instinctual impulse towards masturbation is quite strong. The consequences of surrendering to this instinctual pleasure, however, are colored with feelings of guilt and self-loathing. These feelings in turn cause anxiety and frustration, which build until they require relief. The most convenient relief is to masturbate once again. According to Freud, this cycle of increase and reduction of anxiety is paralleled in all addictive behaviors. Levin (1987) explains that in Freud's view,

> ... masturbation is the 'model' addiction, upon which all later addictions are based. Substance addictions are substitutes for and re-enactment of the addiction to masturbation. (p. 75)

Abraham (1908), an early psychoanalyst, studied the relationship between sexuality and alcohol use. Abraham followed Freud's ideas on psychosexual phases and explored character formation according to fixations at different levels of psychosexual development. Thus, psychoanalytic literature contains references to oral, anal, phallic, and genital character organizations. Since the early days of psychoanalysis there have been approaches other than these for understanding character formation. For example, the character can be understood via the defensive organization or through the level of self and object integration. Nevertheless, Abraham's classic descriptions of the oral, anal, phallic, and genital characters remain useful. The clinical evidence still validates the use of Abraham's conceptualization of character formation despite the fact that there are now other useful ways of looking at character formation and organization.

Abraham's conceptualization of the oral character is especially important for understanding the character of the drug user. During the first year of life, the infant's needs, perceptions, and modes of expression are mainly centered around the mouth, the lips, the tongue, the pharynx and the upper digestive system. The infant's feelings of pleasure (and aggression) originate in these bodily areas, called the oral zone, and organize the psyche. When oral expressions are blocked, oral conflicts ensue. These conflicts may manifest in excessive eating, vomiting, jaw spasms, or in mental patterns like optimism, pessimism, excessive generosity, or dependency. Abraham viewed drug use as a result of an oral conflict, conceptualizing alcoholism as an oral regressive and homoerotic tendency (Levin, 1987). Abraham arrived at this conclusion after observing that men were more openly and physically affectionate with each other when drinking in a bar. In Abraham's mind, alcohol allowed the expression of repressed homosexual urges. Hence, alcoholics were seen to have conflicts related to homosexuality as well as problems that caused them to regress to an infantile oral state. [Socarides (1974) has also linked homosexuality to compulsive drug use, as will be discussed later).]

One of the earliest psychoanalytic papers dealing specifically with drug use pathology was written by Rado (1933). Following along an obvious psychoanalytic line of reasoning, Rado claimed that drug use represented an attempt to regress to a blissful infantile state. Drug use was conceptualized as symptom specific, with specific psychopathology underlying the use of a drugs. Drug users were said to suffer from pathological states of depression, low pain tolerance, and omnipotent narcissism. The effects of drugs were seen as essentially orgasmic. An increase in drug use, however, was thought to be accompanied by a decrease in genital potency. Involvement with drugs was also seen as an abandonment of object relations.

Glover (1939) believed that drug users were at a level of pathology that was between neurotic and psychotic. This was thought of as a new set of transitional pathologies. This new level of pathology was seen as more resistant than neuroses, but neither as a psychotic or borderline state. Glover also affirmed the importance of the aggressive drive in drug addicts, which has the effect of masking guilt. Finally, drugs were seen as objects with the loving and hating characteristics of both parents, a point of view which will be amplified in the next chapter.

Although Fenichel does not really belong to the older psychoanalytic circle, he is included in this section because more than anyone else, he has summarized the ideas of classical psychoanalysis. Fenichel (1945) conceptualized drug use along the lines of Rado, especially with regards to the regression to early infantile oral states. According to Fenichel, these states resulted in oral dependency and depression among alcoholics. Alcoholism was seen as a defense against neurotic conflicts related to dependency and anger. Fenichel recognized that alcohol 'dissolves' inhibitions and rigid defenses (i.e., the superego). He also saw drug use as an attempt at self-medication.

Some writers maintain that many of these early psycho-analytic ideas are outmoded and of little more than anecdotal use to the practicing clinician today. This is especially true with regards to the emphasis on the regressive wish-fulfilling aspects of drugs (DeAngelis, 1975; Wurmser, 1974). However, it can be argued that the older psychoanalytic literature on drug use and addiction should be evaluated according to the history of psychoanalysis. Freud's discovery of the oedipus complex and infantile sexuality necessarily made him pay more attention to a comparison of masturbation and addiction. With the investigation of orality and oral character formation, compulsive drug use was simply explained as a regression to, and fixation at, the oral phase of psychosexual development. These ideas still have validity today. Some of these early ideas, with some modifications, found their ways into more modern ideas about compulsive drug use. For example, Glover's bringing our attention to the aggressive drive echoes its role in the current idea that compulsive drug users function at the level of borderline personality organization. Other early ideas, especially regarding the basic depressive character of opiate addicts, narcissism and object relations deficits, also seem applicable today (Fine, 1972). For a thorough review of the early literature on drug use pathology, see H. Rosenfeld (1965) and Wurmser (1978).

Manic Depression and Compulsive Drug Use

An intriguing psychoanalytic view of drug use pathology was described by Federn (1952). In his writing Federn calls attention to the similarities between the drug addict and those who suffer from manic states. Both the manic and the addict attempt to avoid the possibility of frustration. Neither the manic nor the drug addict can tolerate frustration and both are left impotent in its presence. This frustration is the product of the inability to satisfy cravings for mental pleasure. As Federn (1952) says,

> No addict can stand his craving for satisfaction for any
> length of time. While the manic is able to shift his crav-

> ing for mental pleasure from one object to another, the
> addict is chained to his specific addiction. When it is
> frustrated he must do everything he can to obtain satis-
> faction or else he succumbs to the greatest despair, and
> to a suicidal state of panic. (p. 276)

Addiction is also seen by Federn as an avoidance of depression, which is another by-product of the inability to tolerate frustration. This idea is supported by the fact that
many addicts become depressed when their addiction is
cured. In other words, a state of depression underlies addictive pathology in the same way it underlies mania.
Addiction is seen as an intermediate between mania and depression. A manic person who can no longer maintain the
flight of thoughts necessary for mania will lapse into a state
of impulsiveness, which Federn likens to an addiction. When
the impulsive addiction can no longer be maintained, depression occurs. The reverse is also true. A manic-depressive
individual may seek the intermediate impulsive-addictive
state to avoid swinging between mania and depression. The
genesis of an addiction may, therefore, begin as an escape
from the extremes of a manic-depressive illness. Once the
addiction is alleviated, maintaining a balance between mania
and depression becomes the central concern. This balance
can only be maintained through the tolerance of "mental
pain". Manics, depressives, manic-depressives and addicts
suffer from a deficiency in their ability to tolerate mental
pain, specifically, ego pain. In treatment, the ego's inability
to tolerate mental pain needs to be confronted, or as Federn
(1952) says,

> Whoever wants to remain mentally sound should stand
> a good deal of the pain of frustration, or of the despair
> created through the loss of an object, before he begins to
> compensate for the loss and to master the pain. (p. 278).

For Federn, therefore, the treatment of the compulsive
drug user should be geared towards helping him tolerate his
mental suffering without the refuge of either a drug or
manic-depressive illness. As shall later be elucidated, the
loss of an early object may be one of the keys to understand-

ing why the compulsive drug user cannot tolerate pain and frustration.

Preoedipal Conditions and Compulsive Drug Use

Psychopathy

Arieti (1967) relates the characteristics of the drug addict to the simple psychopath. The drug addict, like the psychopath, experiences tension, physical discomfort, anxiety, pain and a general malaise. The drug addict "...gives the impression of mainly wanting to remove unpleasure" (Arieti, 1967, p. 263). The addict, however, differs from the psychopath in his ability to be aware of his anxiety, sense of defeat and insecurity. He is often conscious of his anxiety, hostility and lack of impulse control, as well as his unstable childhood and dysfunctional personal history. The addict deals with all these problems by transforming them into the struggle to obtain the drug. Rather than escaping reality through a psychotic break, the drug addict deals with reality by reducing it into a search for drugs. Psychotherapy is very difficult for the drug addict because a rational treatment is self-defeating. A more constructive approach would be a therapeutic course that will help the addict tolerate anxiety so that he can receive and maintain the warm approval and deep concern of the therapist. The addict also differs from the alcoholic, who drinks in order to release inhibitions and become aggressive, vindictive and grandiose.

Sexual Deviations

Socarides (1974) has linked homosexuality with drug addiction. In his view both preoedipal-type homosexuals[1]

---

[1]It is important to distinguish between homosexuality as a lifestyle choice and a compulsive homosexuality related to a psychopathological condition. Socarides is referring to the latter, which he terms preoedipal. The comments made here are not meant as a negative description of homosexuals in general. Instead this text seeks to address the problems of individuals who must compulsively engage in certain behaviors. Many different behaviors can become destructive or pathological. These behaviors include eating, heterosexual acts, homosexual acts, etc. Society does not pronounce that eating is bad because of the existence of

and drug addicts suffer from similar preoedipal pathology which is related to anxiety from early childhood. Both the use of drugs and the homosexual act are reparative, providing a 'magical' external solution to the threat of self-annihilation. As Socarides (1974) says,

> The homosexual act itself may be likened to the effects of the opium alkaloids in their magical restorative powers: the optimum "fix", reinstating the body ego and sense of self against a threat of disruption, and in severe cases, imminent disintegration of the personality. (p. 301)

Both preoedipal homosexuality and drug use pathology have seemingly different clinical pictures on the surface. However, the underlying personality organizations in both seem to be the same, requiring a fix, (either a drug or the performance of a homosexual act) "...to maintain the equilibrium of a highly disturbed individual" (Socarides, 1974, p. 300). Freud (1926) spoke of anxiety as having primacy over all other affects. Socarides findings suggest that sexual deviations, which are defined as obligatory ritualized acts in order to reach orgasm, respond to the suffering produced not only by anxiety, but also the painful affect of depression. As Socarides (1985) suggests,

> The pervert attempts to regain his capacity for pleasure and the enjoyment of life by spurious means, bringing about the illusion of control through the magical powers of seduction and sensuality. His triumph lifts him to a state of intoxication, euphoria, and even elation. Elsewhere, I have termed the homosexual's reintegration through incorporation of another man's body and his phallus as the 'optimal fix' (Socarides, 1968), resembling the experience following the intake of opium derivatives, restoring body ego boundaries, and producing a sense of well-being and temporary integration. (p. 332)

Psychotic and Borderline Disorders
Based on his experience in treating nearly a thousand patients, Wurmser (1974) outlined a number of causes and

---

anorexics. Likewise, homosexuality should not be negatively judged because some homosexual behavior derives from a psychopathological condition.

psychodynamic factors related to drug use. Wurmser characterizes drug use as symptomatic of deeper psychological problems. He claims that if a drug is removed from a user they will substitute other symptoms. These other symptoms include neurotic depression, suicide attempts, violent acts, stealing, anxiety attacks, etc. Wurmser suggests that any of these symptoms, which are found prior to the use of drugs, can reappear in a much stronger form when the use of drugs is halted. It is often the case that the reappearance of these symptoms is more dangerous than the drug use itself.

From his observations, Wurmser believes that most compulsive drug users suffer from borderline or psychotic states. " I have never yet seen a compulsive drug user who has not been emotionally deeply disturbed, who has not shown in his history the ravages of borderline, or even psychotic conflicts and defects" (p. 824). This viewpoint is in contradiction to some recent research (Blatt, Berman, et al., 1984), but is in agreement with other analytic writers (Kernberg, 1975), most notably those from France and Italy (Callea & Rubino, 1980; Charles-Nicolas, Valleur & Tonnelier, 1982).

The psychopathology of the compulsive drug user is thought to stem from massive narcissistic disturbances which arise from family pathology. As Wurmser says,

> Parents who did not provide a minimum of consistency, of reliability, of trustworthiness, of responsiveness to the child, especially during his developmental crises, are not usable as inner beacons; instead they become targets of rebellious rage and disdain. Parents who vacillate between temper tantrums and indulgence, who allow themselves to live out their most primitive demands...cannot impart the important combination of love and firmness...(Wurmser, 1974, p. 836)

In this view it is a narcissistic crisis which compels an individual to seek out drugs in an addictive fashion. By 'narcissistic crisis' what is meant is a loss of self-esteem and self-love which produces strong feelings of anxiety. Drugs provide a sense of control of psychic life for the user. This control relieves the anxiety caused by the narcissistic crisis and its attendant overwhelming affect. All drug use, for Wurmser, therefore, is an attempt at self-treatment. This self-treatment varies depending on the affects engendered by the narcissistic conflict. Narcotics and depressant drugs are used to calm intense feelings of rage, hostility, shame, guilt and loneliness. Psychedelic drugs, on the other hand, are understood as counteracting an emotional state of emptiness, boredom and meaninglessness. These drugs are used an antidote to a pervasive feeling of disillusionment or ennui. Stimulants such as amphetamines and cocaine are understood to be similar in effect to the psychedelics. However, Wurmser also sees the stimulants as imparting a sense of aggressive mastery, control, and grandiosity which serve as defenses against massive depression and feelings of unworthiness and weakness. Serious decompensation can occur if abstinence from these various forms of self-medication is attempted without supporting the drug user's ego and sense of self-esteem.

Kernberg (1975) has conceptualized compulsive drug users as suffering from borderline personality organization. According to Kernberg borderline patients are not psychotic in that they do not fuse their self-representations with object representations. Psychotic individuals have diffuse, weak ego structures. Borderline individuals, on the other hand, have egos that can generally conduct reality testing in all but a few specific areas. These areas of weak ego functioning are usually related to interpersonal relationships. Although the egos of borderline individuals are reasonably cohesive, they employ primitive defensive mechanisms, which are usually not found in neurotic individuals. These defenses include *splitting, projective identification* and *denial in the service of splitting*. Narcissistic defenses such as *mirroring, idealization, omnipotence* and *devaluing* are also commonly used by the borderline individual. In Kernberg's view, borderline personality organization encompasses a wide range of pathology. The most primitive borderline individuals are characterized by hostile paranoid features combined with a high degree of impulsively and rage. Higher functioning borderline individuals display many of the characteristics of pathological narcissism.

Kernberg's ideas attempt to provide a bridge between the view that holds object investment secondary to the expression of drives and that which stresses the primacy of the infant's attachment to the object. Furthermore, Kernberg states that the borderline individual is between the level of the neurotic and the psychotic. What is meant is that the borderline individual's ego is more cohesive than the psychotic's and less cohesive than the neurotic's. A more exact way of looking at borderline personality disorder is to assess it from the view of developmental object relations. Although this foreshadows the next chapter, it will be useful to describe the borderline individual in these terms here.

Kernberg (1967, 1975), V. Volkan (1976, 1987) and Searles (1986) have precisely delineated borderline personality organization as a clinical entity by describing the constellation of the borderline individual's self and object representations. An object in this sense can be defined as a mental representation of another person or thing. *Good* object representations are libidinally invested and *bad* object representations are aggressively invested. Rather than just looking at an individual's level of ego organization, Kernberg (1975) examines both the individual's ability to differentiate between self and object representations, and integrate good and bad object representations. The differentiation between self and object representations is a sign of a cohesive sense of self, while the ability to integrate good and bad object representations is a crucial developmental step towards a healthy personality. Within this developmental scheme then, neurotic individuals are seen as having a cohesive sense of self and integrated good and bad object representations. More primitive individuals, such as psychotics have neither a cohesive sense of self or integrated object representations. Borderline individuals have a coherent sense of self but are unable to integrate good and bad object representations.

The inability to integrate good and bad object, and self-representations leads to the quality of splitting which is so characteristic of the borderline individual. During the early development of the child there is a period of normal splitting between good and bad object representations which are invested with libidinal and aggressive drives. Because the growing child's ego is not fully developed, it is not yet able to integrate self and object representations. Other factors, both genetic and biological, can also influence the development of the child's ability to outgrow this stage of splitting. Of course, psychological trauma can have great negative impact on the child's ability to integrate object representations. Too much pre-genital aggression, by itself, can cause psychological trauma and prevent integration. However, the inability to integrate good and bad object representations can usually be traced to an overt trauma such as rape (Katan, 1973), contradictory parenting (Searles, 1986; V. Volkan, 1987), loss of a parent (Furman, 1986), and incest (P. Kernberg, 1989). Other, more subtle features of the family environment can also have a negative effect upon the child's ability to integrate good and bad object representations. (V. Volkan, 1987).

When a child is unable to develop to the point where it is able to integrate good and bad object representations, the splitting of good and bad object representations becomes a dominant defense mechanism and the child's capacity for integration is stunted. Defensive splitting, along with denial, omnipotence, devaluation of self and others, idealization, introjection and projection are used to maintain opposing identifications based upon aggressively tinged bad object representations and libidinally tinged good object representations. These good and bad object representations are alternatively projected and introjected. This prevents the development of an ego identity as described by Erikson (1956). Therefore, although borderline individuals maintain relatively good reality testing, they also demonstrate many areas of ego weakness such as lack of impulse control, acting out, poor tolerance of frustration, etc.

There are many similarities between borderline individuals and compulsive drug users. Like borderline individuals, compulsive drug users often have relatively good reality testing and ego strength. Indeed, it would be very difficult for a drug addict to obtain drugs (a complex interaction with his external reality) without some good localized reality testing. Compulsive drug users, like borderline individuals, also tend to have severe deficits in the ability to participate in interpersonal relationships. The etiology of both borderline and compulsive drug use pathology points to early object trauma. (This will be more fully elucidated in the next chapter.) In general, it is possible to conclude that both borderline individuals and compulsive drug users seek to experience a relationship with a good parent. They also seek to compensate for the experience of bad parenting, or the trauma caused by a parent. In Kernberg's view, compulsive drug use can be thought of as another defensive tactic of the borderline individual. Drug use, in this sense, serves to keep the good and bad object representations apart, preserving the all-good object representation by splitting it off from the all-bad object representation. For Kernberg, the prognosis of treatment with borderline drug users is related to the presence of narcissistic personality structures, impulse control, the ability to use an external structure to suppress addiction, and antisocial behavior. While the ability to control impulses, ask for help and avoid antisocial behavior are indicative of a positive prognosis, the presence of narcissistic structures is indicative of a negative outcome.

A narcissistic personality structure is similar to that of the borderline except that there is a pathological formation of the self-representation called a *grandiose self*. Narcissistic individuals, like borderline individuals, may have had a traumatic childhood. However, their parent or caretaker sees an element in the child which is supported or reinforced in order to compensate for the psychological deficiency of the parent. For example, the mother may think that the developing child will grow up and assure the family's fame or fortune. The parent's unconscious grandiose fantasy about the child becomes part and parcel of the developing child's self-system. A typical narcissistic individual is capable of carrying on their life by pumping his grandiose self from day to day. In narcissistic individuals drug use supports the grandiose self. According to Kernberg the presence of narcissistic personality structures are indicative of a negative prognosis as the drug "...may constitute a mechanism to 'refuel' the pathological grandiose self and assure its omnipotence and protection against a potentially frustrating and hostile environment in which gratification and admiration are not forthcoming" (Kernberg, 1975, p. 222).

According to Kernberg, it is important to set strict rules before treatment can proceed. For suicidal and drug-using

borderline patients, Kernberg asks that they control and assume responsibility for their impulses. If the impulse towards suicide, drug use, or other antisocial behavior cannot
be controlled, the patient must be able to get external help
(from someone besides the analyst or psychoanalytic therapist) if the treatment is to continue. This external help allows
the therapist to maintain his analytic stance so that he or she
does not have to provide a more supportive approach to
therapy.

D. Rosenfeld (1976, 1992, 1993) also understands compulsive drug use as a borderline-level phenomenon, although he tends to conceptualize the addict more toward the
psychotic end of the borderline spectrum. In Rosenfeld's
view (which follows the theories of Melanie Klein), Good
and bad objects are split in order to protect the good object
representation from the primitive envy embodied in the bad
object representation. This splitting arises from the infant's
experience with his mother or primary caretaker who has
fantasies about the child which are inconsistent with her
ability to tolerate his needs. This leads to the existence of
'bad' and 'good' mother object representations. The primitive envy of the bad mother object representation threatens
to destroy the good mother object representation. By keeping
these object representations split, the good mother object
representation is protected. Drugs help to maintain this split
by alternatively (and never simultaneously) representing
both the negative aspects of the bad mother and the positive
sensations of the good mother, without integration.

Rosenfeld describes five stages in the psychoanalytic
treatment of compulsive drug users. In the first stage the
drug using patient takes drugs indiscriminately and acts out
in perverse and promiscuous ways. The patient may become
suicidal and paranoid. It is important during the first stage
for any interpretations to elucidate the distinctiveness between therapist and patient. In the second stage the patient
begins to use one type of drug to the exclusion of all others.
The patient often divides drugs into 'good' and 'bad', with
the bad drugs having a persecutory tinge. During the third
stage the patient becomes increasingly dependent upon the
therapist and the therapy hour. The patient has an especially

difficult time when the therapist is not available, for instance on the weekends. At the fourth stage the patient may tentatively stop using the drug. The patient may also begin to use other material objects, such as cultural or artistic objects as a substitute for the drug. These objects are treated almost like fetishes and can often be used in a compulsive fashion. The patient may also become depressed and suicidal during this stage. In the fifth stage the patient is clinically more neurotic. He can tolerate both the good and bad aspects of the therapy and even internalize some of the good aspects. The patient becomes less grandiose and his life plans become more realistic. The therapist is increasingly seen as a separate individual.

Rosenfeld points out that these stages are not fixed. Often positive changes in the patient's psychopathology will be followed by periods of regression and entrenchment. Therapeutic evolution and regression can occur simultaneously.

Rosenfeld also comments that drug use, especially the intravenous variety, serves to remind the addict that their body exists and that it is filled with fluids, viscera, etc. This type of drug use may be indicative of a psychotic body image, in which the addict feels that his or her body is empty. As Rosenfeld explains,

> Neither the idea of the erogenous zone nor that of the skin as a body limit exists in these patients, but only the notion of a body full or empty of such liquids. hence their need to inject themselves. (1992, p. 236)

The idea of the addict lacking a skin or a body boundary is also important in understanding the addict who,

> ...is attempting to achieve unity through a very precarious organizer, that is, a drug that functions as a poor-quality paste or glue but represents a real striving to find something which will provide a structure. (1992, p. 241)

In his later work Rosenfeld (1992) conceptualizes three categories of drug users, Category A, most easily identifiable in the above discussion, is a person who needs to use a drug to create a container for the body like a skin. These drugs users usually have suffered some type of object loss. If they are treated early and accept the treatment, they have a good prognosis for recovery. Category B drug addicts search for powerful stimuli so they can feel alive and not confuse themselves with dead objects. These addicts may overdose or act out suicidal fantasies. The prognosis varies for these addicts, but they usually accept treatment. Nevertheless, Rosenfeld reports that this is a difficult type of addict to work with and they often drop out of treatment. Category C addicts seek to obtain very primitive body/feeling sensations, which they feel are necessary for their survival. These addicts feel that if they cannot obtain a drug they will lose their identity and disappear. The prognosis for treatment with this type of addict is poor.

Drug Use, Neurotic Pathology and Defenses

Edelstein (1975) has characterized a number of factors related to the compulsive drug user which indicate both a regressed character and a severe neurosis. These factors include early developmental defects, low stimulus barriers, object relations deficits, separation-individuation disturbances, perceptual problems, dedifferentiation of affect and the inability to anticipate or tolerate tension. These problems point to the compulsive drug user as an oral, regressed character. Nevertheless, Edelstein elaborates on the apparently neurotic adaptive mechanisms used by these drug users. These adaptive mechanisms usually consist of repetitive-compulsive behaviors which may take many forms or styles. The simplest form of repetition-compulsion is the compulsion to use drugs because of the inability to postpone satisfaction or tolerate frustration. Drug-taking induces experiences that avoid this type of frustration. When the drug wears off, the frustration and the tension return along with the need to avoid these affects. The next level of repetition-compulsion includes an attempt to induce or change an affect which is usually passively experienced by the drug user. The induction or change of the affect in an active fashion represents control over it. In drug users this change or induction of affect is, not surprisingly, accomplished by way of a drug. The changes caused by the drug are once again temporary, so that the drug must be used again in order for the user to recapture the feelings of control and mastery. The final mechanism is somewhat more elaborate than the previous ones. This mechanism is a combination of wish-fulfilling and control mechanisms. The drug user takes a drug in response to conditions outlined in the above mechanisms. At the same time, due to the superego, the drug user is extremely self-critical and hateful to himself. This, of course, creates more intolerable affect which must be avoided or changed. The addition of further intolerable affect into the system serves to perpetuate the cycle of drug use.

In his later writings, Wurmser (1978, 1985, 1987), has mediated his description of the psychodynamics of compulsive drug use. Rather than conceptualizing drug users as borderlines or psychotics, Wurmser now understands these patients to be suffering from severe neuroses, although these neurotic conflicts are different in nature than those experienced by most neurotics. A key concept in Wurmser's reconceptualization of drug use pathology is the existence of a phobic core structure that underlies the anxiety and dysphoria seen in compulsive drug users. These phobic symptoms and characteristics are related to a defense against overbearing superego functions. Wurmser (1978, 1985) describes a typical sequence of dynamic events in the compulsive drug user. The first stage is a severe inner (superego) pressure or criticism. The second stage is a 'fantastic' feeling after some sort of success is achieved. The third stage is a 'trance' or altered state of consciousness which has a sudden unaccountable onset. This trance is accompanied by intense feelings of loneliness, being unloved, humiliated, guilt or shame and paralyzing panic. The fourth stage is an impulsive attempt to gain relief through the use of drugs. The fifth stage is a suicidal depression accompanied by calls for help, feelings of contrition and self-criticism. The sixth stage is a 'point of relaxation' accompanied by a feeling that 'all is forgiven'. The drug user tries to be good and comply, but in doing so he once again begins to submit to the inner judge of his superego, re-initializing the cycle.

At various points in this cycle, different aspects of the superego hold sway, leading to what Wurmser terms a 'split identity' or a pattern of multiple personalities. If the cycle is severe enough to cause a loss of perceptual reality, "it is as if the patient were possessed: a demon takes over" (1987, p. 160). (This state of possession will be examined in the context of the object relations of the compulsive drug user in the next chapter.) In the severe neurosis of the compulsive drug user, defenses such as denial and splitting are prevalent. In many cases these defenses are used against conflicts which are oedipal in nature.

Blatt and his colleagues (Blatt, Berman, Bloom-Feschbach, Sugarman, Wilber & Kleber, 1984; Blatt, McDonald, Sugarman & Wilber, 1984; Blatt, Rounsaville, Eyre & Wilber, 1984) have extensively studied opiate addicts and polydrug abusers from a psychoanalytic perspective. These studies have applied a rigorous quasi-experimental and statistical methodology (Campbell & Stanley, 1963; Sarnoff, 1971) to the examination of psychodynamic hypotheses.

As previously indicated, many psychoanalytic theorists believe that opiate addicts function at a very primitive level of personality organization (narcissistic, psychotic, or borderline psychology). According to Blatt,

> ...opiate addiction has been conceptualized as a regressive phenomenon in which the addict seeks immediate pleasure and satisfaction in an intense, symbiotic state either as compensation for profound early deprivation or to recapture an overindulged, infantile state, as a defense against the threat of psychotic disintegration, or as a retreat from painful neurotic affects such as depression and anxiety which result from frustrations and disappointments in interpersonal relations. (Blatt, Berman, et al., 1984, p. 157)

Using a number of standardized personality measures, Blatt and his co-workers decided to test this assumption. The *Bellack Ego Functions Interview*, the *Loevinger Sentence Completion*, and the *Rorschach* were used to evaluate the degree and nature of psychopathology among 99 opiate addicts and to compare them with normal and mentally ill groups. Results indicated that the addicts were not suffering from thought-disorder or deficient reality testing when compared to psychiatric patients. The addicts did, however, have significant impairment in their developmental level of object relations and their ability to control their affect when compared to the psychiatric patients. It was concluded that opiate addicts do not have problems in their cognitive functioning, but instead have difficulty in establishing meaningful and satisfying interpersonal relationships. This was seen as indicative that opiate addicts seeking treatment suffer from a neurotic level pathology characterized by depression and the inability to moderate their emotions. Opiate addicts were not thought of as suffering from a more primitive level of pathology as has been previously thought in psychoanalytic circles. In Blatt's concept, opiate addicts have selected "...an isolated mode for achieving the satisfactions and pleasures most people seek in interpersonal relationships" (Blatt, Berman, et al., 1984, p. 163).

In another study, Blatt, Rounsaville, et al. (1984), further elucidated the nature of psychopathology among opiate addicts. Once again these addicts were compared to clinical and non-clinical populations. Additionally, a group of non-addicted, polydrug abusers were included in the comparison. In this study the groups were compared using standardized measures of depression. As outlined above, a number of previous studies have indicated that opiate addicts suffer from a primitive depressive pathology.

There are two conceptualizations of depression in psychoanalytic theory, *anaclitic* and *introjective*. Anaclitic depression is derived from intense fears of abandonment and the desperate need to maintain contact with a gratifying object. Anaclitic depression was first described by Spitz (1946). The word anaclitic signifies dependence upon others. Spitz described a syndrome among infants and children consisting of apprehension, weeping, withdrawal, sadness, and refusal to eat or relate to others. The infants studied by Spitz were around nine months of age. He found that anaclitic depression resulted if the mothers of the infants were absent for at least three months.

Introjective depression refers to a lowering of self-esteem after a loss. In this situation, loss of an object is tantamount to loss of part of the self-image. Introjective depression, therefore, engenders feelings of worthlessness, self-criticism, shame, guilt and idealized parental standards which stem from the internalization of harsh parental objects (superego). Anaclitic depression is understood as being developmentally inferior and more primitive than introjective depression. It should be mentioned that there is some controversy over the distinctions between anaclitic and introjective depression. Some writers like Beres (1966) maintain that all depression is related to superego conflicts and that the symptoms of both anaclitic and introjective depression outlined above can be explained as a result of such conflicts. Nevertheless, the levels of personality organization for each set of symptoms—primitive for anaclitic symptoms and more advanced for introjective symptoms—still holds. Therefore, for the purpose of studying compulsive drug use, the distinctions between anaclitic and introjective depression are valid.

Because opiate addicts have been characterized as suffering from primitive psychopathology, their depression has been commonly thought of as anaclitic. After discovering that opiate addicts suffer from a neurotic level dysfunction, Blatt and his colleagues (Blatt, Rounsaville, et al., 1984; Blatt, McDonald, et al., 1984) suspected that addicts did not suffer from the more primitive anaclitic depression, but from introjective depression. As they put it,

> ...addiction is not considered as an anaclitic seeking of the immediate gratification of a mindless, trouble-free state to replace oral deprivation and feelings of neglect, but as withdrawal and isolation from human relationships because of feelings of low self-esteem and negative expectations in interpersonal interactions. The addict is seen as withdrawn, angry, sullen, empty, hopeless, filled with self-blame and self-loathing...(p. 343)

Using a number of depression-specific measures, including Blatt's *DEQ* scale (Blatt, Quinlan, Chevron, McDonald, & Zuroff, 1982), depression among opiate addicts was characterized in comparison to clinical and non-clinical groups. The results of the study indicated that opiate addicts are more self-critical than either clinical, non-clinical and polydrug abusing groups. Also, among polydrug abusers, there was a relationship between the amount of opiates used and the degree of depression related to self-criticism, which was indicative of introjective depression. It was thought that this may have been an indication that non-addicted drug users who are depressively self-critical are at a greater risk for opiate addiction.

Compulsive Drug Use, Self Psychology and Narcissism

Levin (1987) has outlined an approach tŏ the understanding and treatment of substance abuse based on Kohut's self-psychology (Kohut, 1971, 1977, 1978, 1984). Kohut was a psychoanalyst who developed a variation on both theory and treatment technique after working with patients who suffered from narcissistic personality disorders. These patients did not fit well into pre-existing psychoanalytic theory. They did not seem to possess a sense of self or an identity, yet they were clearly not psychotic or suffering from thought disorders. These patients were also able to establish a strong relationship with their analyst. Nevertheless, the relationship that was established was far from the typical neurotic transference. Instead, these patients developed what Kohut called a "narcissistic transference". In this type of transference, the patient either relates to the analyst as if he were an extension of the patient (mirroring), or as if the patient was part of an omnipotent analyst.

Not surprisingly, Kohut understands addictive behavior as resulting from a narcissistic disturbance. Addiction in this model is seen as a "futile attempt to repair developmental deficits in the self" (Levin, 1987, p. 13). Levin (1987) has applied Kohut's ideas primarily to alcoholics, although he expands this treatment to include other addictions as well. He conceptualizes alcoholics as suffering from four types of pathology. Alcoholics are seen as self-destructive, lacking self components responsible for self-care and self-esteem, overly self-involved, and as having a fragile sense of self or identity.

While theoretically, Levin's use of Kohut's approach is in strong agreement with psychoanalytic thought, it differs radically with regard to treatment technique. For Levin (1987), "The therapist must diagnose, confront and educate" (p 92). In other words, the technical neutrality of the therapist must be modified to treat substance abusers. Levin goes on to say,

> On one hand, some analytically oriented practitioners attempt to maintain a stance of "technical neutrality" when what is needed is an active stance that the patient cannot improve until the drinking stops. (p. 92)

This approach to treatment is fundamentally at odds with the classical psychoanalytic method (Fine, 1972), although psychoanalysts have been known to require that prospective patients seek detoxification or inpatient care before beginning analysis (Kernberg, 1975; H. Rosenfeld, 1965; Wurmser, 1985). Wurmser (1985), in contrast, expounds a modern analytic stance to the drug using patient,

> It has been my experience that it is better *not* to be placed into such a role of punisher and warner. A consistently analytic approach can be more effective if it remains grounded in, and compatible with a *strong emotional presence* of the therapist, an attitude of warmth, kindness, and flexibility. (p. 94).

Levin (1987) recognizes that confronting and educating the patient will be difficult for the therapist. Overcoming this difficulty relies on the ability of the therapist to establish a strong relationship (transference) with the patient before undertaking confrontational and didactic roles. This strong relationship will slowly allow the therapist to be substituted for the drug. On this point the Kohutian and psychoanalytic approaches are in agreement. These issues will be covered in more depth in the section on treatment.

Dodes (1990) extends many of the narcissistic characteristics described above to compulsive drug users of all types. He conceptualizes the roles of power, helplessness and rage as being central to the psychodynamics of addiction. Dodes sees drug use as a mechanism which provides an omnipotent control over the drug user's affective state. This control serves to protect the drug user from being flooded by helplessness or powerlessness. Dodes also sees drug use as the expression of the aggressive drives which coexists with the maintenance of control over feelings of helplessness. The aggressive drives are "in the service of narcissistic equilibrium" and are used "to re-establish the power...which has long been known for its intensity in narcissistically impaired individuals" (p. 414). Dodes terms these drives as "narcissistic rage" which has the same compulsive, insistent qualities as addiction. Addicts use drugs to express narcissistic rage and defend against feelings of powerlessness. They do not, however, necessarily suffer from narcissistic character disorders,

> But most addicts are not narcissistic characters. The shame that may be associated with anal and separation-individuation/autonomy issues, or narcissistic injuries associated with oedipal impotence, guilt, and inhibitions, may all provide the underlying basis for vulnerability to feeling overwhelmed and helpless that is great enough for helplessness to be experienced as a traumatic narcissistic blow. (p. 409)

Dodes' conceptualization of the compulsive drug user remains flexible. The compulsive drug user can be understood as ranging across a continuum of pathology. This flexibility is helpful with regards to the treatment of pathological drug use.

Drug Use, Self-Medication and Dysphoria

Khantzian (1990, 1989, 1987a, 1987b, 1985, 1982, 1980, 1979, 1978, 1974, 1972; Khantzian & Kates, 1978; Khantzian & Treece, 1977) has contributed voluminously to the psychoanalytic understanding of drug dependence. His work presents a number of novel ideas about the relationship of drugs to the psychic life of the individual. Khantzian believes that there is more to the addict's compulsion than a strictly biological mechanism or a psychoanalytic explanation based upon drive theory.

Much of the original psychoanalytic literature from the 1960's and '70s postulates that the first and foremost reason individuals begin to use drugs is to "self-medicate" or to protect themselves against painful or unpleasant affect. This protection also functions as a developmental crutch (Weider & Kaplan, 1969; Krystal & Raskin, 1970; Wurmser, 1974). In an intriguing argument, Khantzian (1974, 1978, 1979) postulates that drugs do not produce euphoria for the addict, but instead provide relief from the *dysphoria* resulting from the addict's rigid, defective or overbearing defenses against affect. Following Krystal and Raskin (1970), Khantzian also believes that different types of patients will use different types of drugs, depending upon the dysphoria experienced. Khantzian proposes three types of drugs users.

The first are the users of narcotics, often described in psychoanalytic literature as attempting to return to a symbiotic, or fused state of object relations. Khantzian believes that narcotic addicts are drawn to the anti-aggressive properties of narcotics to compensate for their own powerful and uncontrollable affect arising from severely defective drive and affect defenses. The second group consists of alcohol and sedative dependent users. This group counters isolation, feelings of coldness; and emptiness through the use of drugs that soften or reduce overly rigid defense mechanisms. The third group consists of stimulant abusers, who use drugs to "...counter states of depletion, anergia, and hyperactivity..." which are associated with "...deflated ego/ego-ideal structures of depressive and narcissistic characters..." (Khantzian, 1987b, p.5).

Khantzian strongly believes that there is a is a dynamic relationship between the suffering produced by a specific drug and the suffering relieved by that drug. He notes that the states associated with physical withdrawal from a specific drug closely resemble the pre-existing painful affect which was originally relieved by the drug. This presents an interesting paradox; that drug use "...often has dual aspects of relieving distress at the same time that the symptom causes suffering in its own right." (1987a, p. 1). From this, Khantzian believes that drug users need to control their affect as much as to relieve themselves from its pain. This control leads to a repetition-compulsion,

> ...repetition and suffering for addicts is not another example...of destructive instincts, masochism or inverted aggression, but probably represents more an attempt to

> control or tolerate suffering which is otherwise experi-
> enced as being beyond a person's control...They actively
> replace preexisting passively experienced admixtures of
> pain, dysphoria, and emptiness with admixtures of
> analgesia, relief, dysphoria and distress produced by the
> drug effects and after effects. (1987, p. 20)

Kernberg (1975) has also concluded that the use of specific drugs are related to specific psychopathologies. For
Kernberg, patients with depressive personalities may use alcohol to achieve a feeling of well-being and euphoria. This is
an attempt to regain a lost parental object whose loss has
created a sense of guilt and depression. As discussed above,
borderline drug users, on the other hand, may use drugs to
keep good and bad objects split from one another. The feeling produced by the drugs allows for the activation of the
good object and the denial of the bad object. This permits an
escape from guilt and internal persecution. Narcissistic borderline patients, as previously mentioned, use drugs to fuel
their sense of grandiosity as a protective response to a hostile
and frustrating environment.

Schiffer (1988) studied the case histories of nine compulsive cocaine users in a framework similar to Khantzian's.
These patients were treated with long-term, in-depth, psychodynamic therapy. The treatment outcome, as reported by
the patients, was successful, with little relapse one year after
the completion of therapy. All of the nine subjects suffered
from disturbed interpersonal and work relationships at the
time of intake and all patients were found to have unrecog-
nized psychological trauma stemming from childhood.
Cocaine addiction was seen as a form of self-medication and
as a repetition-compulsion. The use of cocaine, according to
Schiffer, is "...an unconscious, symbolic repetition of the
early trauma in which old psychological injuries would be
reinflicted by the drug abuser" (1988, p. 133). This re-experience of the early trauma serves to give the drug user a sense
of control over the drug. Hence, cocaine, is important as a
medicine for relieving the unpleasant affect from the original
trauma and is subsequently invested with a great deal of energy. The use of drugs to re-experience past trauma is also
seen by Schiffer not only as an attempt at self-medication,

but also as a self-destructive repetition-compulsion which includes aspects of denial, reaction-formation, and identification with the aggressor.

Summary and Conclusions from the Psychoanalytic Literature

Overall, the above studies indicate that there are many different ways to understand drug use pathology. The modern viewpoints presented in this chapter may be summarized into four categories. The first category includes the writings of Arieti, Federn, Kernberg, D. Rosenfeld, Socarides and Wurmser (1974) and conceptualizes drug use pathology as primitive and preoedipal. Among these authors, the compulsive drug user is seen as manic/depressive, psychopathic, borderline or psychotic. The second category, represented by the writing of Levin and to some degree Dodes, expresses the pathology of the compulsive drug user in terms of narcissistic disturbances as they are understood by Kohut and others. The third category is represented by the work of Khantzian, Edelstein, Schiffer and to some degree Arieti and Dodes. These writers conceptualize the drug user as engaging in an attempt to medicate himself in order to avoid intolerable affect or rage. This self-medication is understood to be a form of repetition-compulsion. Compulsive drug use is also as seen as ranging across a continuum of psychopathology. The fourth category encompasses the work of Wurmser (1978, 1985, 1987) and Blatt in which the compulsive drug user is seen as a severe neurotic who utilizes primitive defense mechanisms and who suffers from phobic and dissociative personality structures or introjective depression.

These apparently contradictory conceptualizations of drug use pathology all contain valid and useful points of view. However, despite the seeming disparity of these points of view, they lead a number of shared conclusions. My first conclusion is that drug use fits into a wide range of psychopathology, although this pathology is circumscribed at the extreme ends of the range. For instance, compulsive drug users do not seem to be psychotic. Although compulsive drug users may be subject to brief reactive psychoses, they do not often present themselves, nor do they permanently regress into, overtly psychotic states. On the other hand, compulsive drug users also do not seem to suffer from simple neuroses, although on first glance their defenses (e.g. denial) may seem to indicate neurotic repression of traumatic material. There is, however, a paradox contained in this conclusion. Although opiate addiction is generally considered the ultimate level of drug use pathology, Blatt's studies indicate that opiate addicts suffer from less primitive pathology than polydrug abusers. Other studies (McLellan, Woody & O'Brien, 1979) have also shown that stimulant and depressive drug abusers are more likely to decompensate into a more primitive level of psychopathology than opiate addicts. Additional work is needed to clarify the range of pathology among opiate addicts and other types of drug abusers. Blatt's studies of opiate addicts may have been misleading in this regard, given that his examination was limited to those addicts who sought help. This group of opiate addicts may be functioning at a much higher level than the addict who remains on the street.

It is possible to see compulsive drug use in any type of personality organization. If a drug user is neurotic the drug will be symbolized at a high level. Compulsive use of drugs at higher levels of personality functioning may be attempts to patch up neurotic conflicts. Nevertheless, it is possible to say that most compulsive drug use pathology falls into the range of what would today be labeled as a borderline pathology, including higher level borderline pathology which presents more like a severe neurosis, borderline pathology with narcissistic features, and more primitive borderline pathology which presents with more psychotic features. In general, it is possible to say that most compulsive drug use would seem to appear in those individuals who have unintegrated self and object representations. In these individuals, drug use helps maintain primitive defense mechanisms like splitting which defend against a psychotic regression. This leads to my second conclusion, that the etiology of the compulsive drug user is based upon early object relations pathology. Another idea, which is present in many of the studies reviewed above, is also related to object relations pathology. This is the presence of hostile, self-critical rage among compulsive drug users. This rage appears to be mitigated or obscured by the effects of drugs.

Indeed, the presence of object relations pathology seems to be the major point on which the studies cited above agree. It is, however, difficult to tell from the above studies whether or not compulsive drug users suffer from an object relations deficit (Kohut), the development of a pathological object relations structure (Kernberg), or both. Part of the confusion here originates in the differing conceptualization of pathological narcissism and borderline personality organization by Kernberg and Kohut. A thorough comparison of these two viewpoints is outlined elsewhere (Adler, 1986) and I will not pursue it here.

Given that compulsive drug users suffer from some sort of preoedipal disturbance and that object relations play an important role in this pathology, it will be useful to examine the relationships of drugs and drug use to object relations. It is quite possible that further study and conceptualization of the constellation of object relations among drug abusers and addicts may resolve some of the different aspects represented in the psychoanalytic literature on drug abuse.

Chapter Four

Object Relations and Compulsive Drug Use

Although drug use has not yet been conceptualized using a purely object relations approach, object relations phenomena are implicit in the psychoanalytic studies outlined in the previous chapter. While these studies of drug use have touched upon the macro-level psychodynamics of drug use, they stop short of explaining these dynamics in detail. The following discussion outlines the concept of object relations and its connection to drug use pathology in more detail.

Object Relations Theory

The ideas underlying object relations theory can be derived from the psychoanalytic drive/structure model, which postulates that the drive energy (libido) seeks *objects* in order to neutralize tension. This tenet is the constancy principle (Freud, 1920), which holds that the basic aim of the psychic apparatus is to maintain stimulation as close as possible to zero. This phenomena can be explained in terms of object relations. The infant is uncomfortable or in a state of tension. When the infant comes into contact with an object, his drive needs are satisfied and his tension is reduced. This tension reduction is associated with pleasure. (Symington, 1986, p. 118)

In order to reduce psychic stimulation and the tension it causes, libido seeks for objects which will neutralize it. These objects share three important properties. First they are always reducible to the underlying drive. Second, objects may include people or things. Third, objects can undergo change.

Objects are not inherent, but are created out of the drive. When the drive is satisfied, or tension reduced, there is an opportunity for the creation of an object, or more accurately, a mental representation of the object. Repeated situations of satisfaction create an internal mental representation of an object from an external situation. In this way an object becomes distinguished from the subject. An object is something (a person or thing) outside of the subject. In psychoanalysis, the term interpersonal relationship is used to indicate the relationship between a subject and an object, while object relations theory is used to describe the relationship between internal representations of objects and the self, within the subject. In other words, object relations theory describes an internal mental representation of an interpersonal relationship. Accordingly, an object relations theory indicates that the mind includes elements taken in from the outside through a process of internalization and that there is an internal relationship between one's self representations and the representation of internalized objects.

Object relations theory is not something outside of classical psychoanalysis. It was included in classical psychoanalysis as a separate focus or point of view. For example, when Freud (1917) described the mental mechanisms at work in the process of mourning he utilized object relations theory. He theorized that when an external object is lost (for instance when a person dies), the shadow (i.e., the mental representation of this person) falls upon the ego of the mourner. When this happens the already existing mental representation of the lost object is re-cathected. This leads to an internal interaction between the representation of the lost object and the representation of the self.

Kernberg (1976) makes a distinction between general and specific approaches to object relations theory. The general approach to object relations theory refers to an understanding of the nature of existing interpersonal relations in terms of past ones. Therefore, in general, object relations theory seeks to understand how past object relations are internalized and become psychic structures. These past object relations are seen as determining, to a great extent, the current nature of the interaction between the subject and his objects. As Kernberg (1976) says,

> Psychoanalytic object relation theory, at this level, represents a general focus or approach occupying an intermediate field between psychoanalytic metapsychology proper, on the one hand, and clinical analyses of normal and pathological functioning on the other. (p. xiii-xiv)

The more specific view of object relations theory refers to the building up of dyadic intrapsychic representations of self and object images. Such representations reflect the original relationship between the infant and its primary object (usually the mother or primary caretaker). These relationships are later elaborated into triadic and multiple internal and external interpersonal relationships. This way of understanding object relations theory has been greatly refined by Kernberg (1967, 1975, 1980) who synthesized the works of Bowlby, Erikson, Fairbairn, Jacobson, Klein, and Mahler.

In both the general and specific models of object relations theory there is a strong developmental thrust: The infant originally relates only to himself to satisfy his drive needs. As he ages, he begins to receive satisfaction from relationships to objects outside or external to himself. The first and primary object is usually the mother, or a part of the mother (e.g. the breast). This relationship to the primary object becomes the prototype of all relationships for the rest of the infant's life. Consequently, disturbances in this relationship have profound and far-reaching effects upon the infant's mental health.

A number of different theorists have elaborated upon the development of object relationships (Blanck & Blanck, 1986; Jacobson, 1964; Kernberg, 1975, 1980; Mahler, 1975). The developmental models outlined by these authors tend to follow Freud's initial ideas about object relations closely. Nevertheless, these modern authors emphasize different stages of the developmental path. The most common concep-

tualization of the stages of object relations development are
as follows;

1. *Infantile Autism*—This is the beginning stage which is
   similar to Freud's idea of primary narcissism in which
   the infant has not yet developed the ability to perceive or
   acknowledge anything external to himself. Much psychoanalytic research has been conducted on the beginning of mentation among infants (Emde, 1985;
   Greenspan, 1989; Stern, 1985; Tähkä, 1988). This research
   indicates that the infant's mind is more active than previously thought. There are potentials of mental functions,
   including relations to objects. Some mental function potentials get activated through more complicated relationships that exist between infant and the mother. These
   findings indicate that the concept of autism should be reconsidered. It may be better to talk about an undifferenti-
   ated state of self and object relations than a completely
   objectless state.

2. *Symbiosis*—In this stage, there is a dawning of external
   reality. There can be no symbiosis if there is no external
   reality. However, the external reality of the infant
   (consisting of its relationship with its mother) is fused
   with its experiences and, therefore, remains undifferenti-
   ated.

3. *Separation-Individuation*—The infant begins to develop a
   sense of separateness from the mother. At first the infant
   can only tolerate this separation for short periods of time,
   but after much practice these time periods lengthen.

4. *Mature Object Relations*—At this stage the infant understands himself to be a separate person from the mother.
   He is able to enter into relationships with the mother and
   others in a way which reflects his understanding that
   they are separate individuals with needs different from
   his.

Each of the developmental stages of object relations represents a progressively more complicated dyadic relationship. Generally speaking, the time period for the unfolding of this developmental pattern is from birth to around three years of age. However, this time period varies widely. Affective states are also tied to the object relations stages. These affective states are originally derived from the biological responses of the infant to the environment and are related to the experience of satisfaction, frustration and panic. It is, therefore, not surprising to find that individuals with object relations pathology often have affective problems as well.

The outcomes of this developmental sequence are healthy psychic structures; ego, superego and id (Kernberg, 1980). The ability to enter into, and resolve triadic relationships such as the oedipal conflict is dependent upon the resolution of object relation conflicts. This is why object relations psychopathology is usually conceptualized as being *preoedipal* in nature. It is important to distinguish preoedipal object relations conflict from other types of conflict at an oedipal level. In classical psychoanalysis oedipal level conflict is described as occurring between unconscious wishes and superego responses. Later on, this type of conflict came to be explained as being related to anxiety. This anxiety is created when expressions of libidinal and aggressive drives come into conflict with both internal and external prohibitions. This conflict is experienced as a form of anxiety which is defended against by the ego. With the systemization of object relations theory within psychoanalysis, conflicts were conceptualized in terms of conflicts among internal self and object representations. In normal development, the child slowly develops an integrated self-representation and integrated object representations. In order to achieve this integration the child needs to gain the ability to put together opposing self and object representations and their drive derivatives. This attempt at integration causes anxiety and conflict. This type of preoedipal, object relations conflict dominate until the child develops a cohesive sense of self and integrated object representations. Once this is achieved, oedipal or structural (id/ego/superego) conflicts become dominant. Dorpat (1976) succinctly describes the difference between structural (oedipal) and object relations (preoedipal) conflict:

> ...in a structural conflict, the subject experiences (or is capable of experiencing if some part of the conflict is unconscious) the opposing tendencies as aspects of himself...in the object relations conflict, the subject experiences the conflict as being between his own wishes and representations (e.g. introjects) of another person's values, prohibitions, or injunctions. (869-870).

Another way of saying this is that if an individual's psychic structure is advanced, he is able to 'own' his conflict, even if aspects of it are unconscious. If the individual's psychic structure has not developed and his internal mental representations are not integrated, he is able to own only part of the conflict while the other part is experienced as if it belongs to someone else.

Drug Use and Object Relations

Drugs have much in common with objects and their representations. They reduce libidinal and aggressive tension and, at least in the short term, give a person a feeling of well-being. This combination of a feeling of well-being and the neutralization of tension makes the drug experience similar to an infantile dependent state, in which the infant is symbiotically related to the primary object. The effects of drugs reduce tension, or in Khantzian's terms, provide relief from dysphoria. It follows that, in general, drug use is regressive in nature, leading the user to seek a return to the experience of this infantile dependent state (Fine, 1972; Rado, 1933). Two aspects of drug use tend to support this idea.

The first is that the drug user tends to be helpless and dependent when he is under the influence of drugs. Although Khantzian states that drugs put the user in control of his dysphoria, it would seem more likely that the drug user alternates between being in control of his dysphoria when the drug effects wear off, and being controlled or 'taken care of', when he is under the influence of the drug.

The second aspect is that the primary model of incorporation of drugs is oral. The mouth is the earliest libidinal zone and of primary importance to drug users. (Miller, 1983, describes a case with an intravenous drug user in which the skin was the primary zone. Although in this case the libidinal zone is different, the basic dynamics of drug use retain their primitive object qualities). These aspects reinforce the idea that drug use represents a return to a state of primitive object relations. This state is characterized by symbiotic dependency on the object, which is experienced as pleasurable, and which provides pleasure primarily through the oral zone (Charles-Nicolas, Valluer & Tonnelier, 1982; Edelstein, 1975). Therefore, although drugs usually carry both good and bad aspects of the early object, individuals with good early object relations are more likely to experience drug use as pleasurable than not. Individuals who had good primary object relations will also be less likely to crave a replay of these early object feelings, having already achieved more stable mature object relations.

For those with disturbed early object relations, drug use may be an attempt to compensate for the ambivalent and frustrating aspects of the primary object, which are characterized by the expression of infantile rage, aggression and confusion. For instance, one study profiled the mothers of frequent drug users as,

> ...relatively cold, unresponsive, and underprotective. They appear to give their children little encouragement while, conjointly, they are pressuring and overly interested in their children's "performance". The apparent net effect of this double-bind is that they turn a potentially enjoyable interaction into a grim and unpleasant one. (Shedler & Block, 1990, p. 621)

It may not only be the primary object (mother) that engenders rage, aggression and confusion in compulsive drug users. Object relations with the father and the family object relation constellation may also play important roles in the etiology of addiction. Wurmser (1978) describes the typical constellation of a family of a drug addict,

> One of the most consistent family constellations identi-
> fied...was the combination of an overprotective indul-
> gent mother with an absent or emotionally distant father.
> Mothers were described as having "special" rela-
> tionships with the sons and tended to be involved in
> their addictions. Some fathers were described as hostile
> and punitive rather than weak and ineffectual, but the
> end result seemed to be that drug addicts did not have a
> role figure with whom to identify in a positive way (p.
> 361).

These dynamics in the etiology of the drug user can be seen clearly in a number of the cases presented later in the text. Of course, the question of specificity is very difficult to address. While the family constellation presented above certainly signal future trouble, an individual with this type of family may not become a compulsive drug user. Instead, he may develop some other type of addiction, sexual perversion, borderline personality disorder, etc.

A negative experience with early or primary objects may cause an individual to crave for the good aspects of these objects throughout his life. This is readily apparent when the primary object failed to provide a sense of security, or when there was a loss of the object. The loss of the object can be real or imagined. For instance, if a mother dies, a real object is lost. If the mother is psychotic, however, there is also a loss of the object in the sense that certain interactions between mother and child will not be available. Without an object an individual may search for experiences which compensate for, or recreate the experience of the good aspects of the early object. The drug experience may play this compensatory role. The research by Blatt and his colleagues (Blatt, Berman, et al., 1984; Blatt, McDonald, et al., 1984; Blatt, Rounsaville, et al., 1984), however, indicates that compulsive drug use may be more than a search for the pleasurable primary object. Instead, it can be understood as an attempt to deal with internalized object representations derived from the negative experience of the primary object. In other words, the harshness and cruelty of the parents, along with the frustration this experience engenders, are introjected and are established as the internal object world of the compulsive drug user. The compulsive use of drugs may be both an attempt to excise and/or control these negative internalized object representations. Therefore, it will be important to examine the object relations dynamics among drug users from the standpoint of a theory that can explain drug use both in terms of regression to the primary object and the internalization of harsh, frustrating object representations.

As noted by Khantzian (1974, 1978, 1979) and Wurmser (1974), different types of drugs may provide different types of compensation. The compensation needed for a particular personality type may be represented by the effects of a particular drug. A study by DeAngelis (1975) examined the relation of client behavior to the type of drug used within the framework of a psychoanalytic treatment milieu. This study supports the idea that personality structures related to specific patterns of object relations are symbiotically drawn to certain drugs due to the reinforcing nature of the drug's effect upon a given object configuration. Another study by Mider (1983) also gives support to this hypothesis. Although little data exists correlating the early object history of drug users with the types of drugs used, it appears likely that clear patterns will emerge.

Drug Use, Bad Objects and Fairbairn's Theory of Object Relations

Thus far, drug use has been examined primarily as a compensation for the good aspects of the primary object. However, the relationship of drug use to the harsh, frustrating or "bad" aspects of the primary object is less clear. In order to describe this relationship it will be useful to examine the object relations theory of W. H. D. Fairbairn.

Fairbairn's major ideas were formulated in two papers, *A Revised Psychopathology of the Psychoses and Psychoneuroses*, and *The Repression and Return of the Bad Objects* (Fairbairn, 1952), both reprinted in Buckley (1986). Although Fairbairn's theories deviate from the psychoanalytic mainstream he is considered to have made important contributions to the field (Kernberg, 1980, 1984). Fairbairn's theory of object relations is helpful in the formulation of a deeper understanding of the psychodynamics of drug use. In fact, the pathology of drug dependence has been characterized in terms of Fairbairn's theories (Callea and Rubino, 1980).

Fairbairn differs from classical psychoanalytic theory in his rejection of the primacy of the drives. Fairbairn believed that objects, and hence object representations, carry libido as opposed to the classical idea that libido seeks objects in order to reduce tension. He also believed that the ego, in at least a rudimentary form, is present from birth. Thus, he did not believe in primary narcissism, postulating instead that narcissistic states were essentially autoerotic, with the infant providing himself with the representation of an object that could not otherwise be obtained. Fairbairn viewed object representations used by the individual in this manner as "...an attempt to compensate by substitutive satisfactions for the failure of his emotional relationships with outer objects" (Fairbairn, 1952, p. 40).

In Fairbairn's view individuals undergo three stages of development. In the first stage the individual is in a state of infantile dependence or identification with the object. This stage is characterized by an attitude of 'taking' or incorporating through the oral zone. The first stage is divided into two parts: the *early oral*, in which the infant relates exclusively to part objects (the breast), and the *late oral*, in which the infant is able to relate to whole objects (the mother).

The next or second stage is that of transition between infantile and mature dependence. During this transition the infant's attitude turns from *taking* to one of *giving*. Objects are split into good and bad representations, with the bad object representations being internalized[1]

---

[1]It is important to note that Fairbairn did not speak of object representations, but only of internalized and externalized objects. For the sake of clarity and consistency with more modern object relations theory, Fairbairn's theories will be explained using modern terminology. That is, *objects* will denote real persons or things, while *object representations* will denote their mental representations. It should also be remembered that although object representations are by definition, internal to the psychic system, they can be internalized, or introjected and externalized, or projected. Regardless of whether or not an object representations is external or internal, it is still a mental representation, whether or not it is projected onto someone or something outside, or internalized and made part of the self-system.

The third stage is that of mature dependence which is characterized by relations to differentiated objects. The attitude is one of *giving*. Both good and bad object representations are externalized.

These theories have a number of applications to drug use, but differ from the classical psychoanalytic explanation in that drugs can be seen as representing bad objects as well as good, or compensatory objects. Drugs, therefore, can represent both primal pleasurable objects and internalized frustrating objects. French analyst, Joyce McDougall (1985) expresses this dynamic eloquently,

> For the enslaved addict, the addictive object—whether it is food, tobacco, alcohol, pharmaceutical products, or opiates—is in the first instance invested as "good", in spite of its sometimes dire consequences...Yet once absorbed, the addictive substance is experienced as bad. (pp. 66-67)

Drug use takes the place of, or compensates for, a satisfying emotional relationship with an external object. This is similar to the psychoanalytic object relations notion of drug use compensating for the experience of the good object. Nevertheless, Fairbairn's theory also gives an indication of the idea that drugs can also serve as representations of bad objects. This conceptualization of drugs as bad object representations explains the underlying self-critical and hostile, introjective pathology found in opiate addicts.

In Fairbairn's theory, bad object representations carry a dual nature as enticing or seductive, and frustrating or rejecting (Cashdan, 1988). These qualities are shared by drugs and can be understood as representing both the 'loving and hating' characteristics of the parents (Glover, 1939). Drugs are exciting or seductive in that they promise to provide pleasure. They are frustrating or rejecting in that, once ingested, this pleasure is short lived and abruptly taken away. The relationship between Fairbairn's theory of object relations and drugs can be understood in the following diagram.

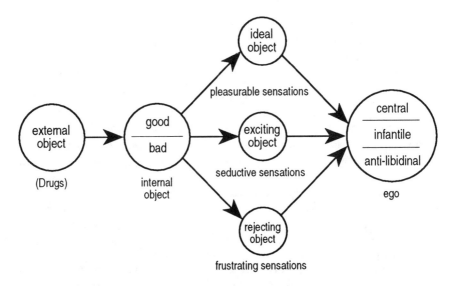

Figure 1. Structural Representation of Fairbairn's Theory of Object Relations with Regards to Drug Use.

In this model representations of external objects are internalized. In an internal state they are split. The good internalized object representation gives rise to the *ideal object,* which in turn becomes integrated into the ego as the *central ego.* The ideal object represents the good and pleasing aspects of a drug.

The bad internal object representation gives rise to two aspects. The first aspect is the *exciting object* which becomes the *infantile ego.* This bad object aspect represents insatiable desire and a promised pleasure which is exciting and seductive. This characterization corresponds well with the drug user's attitude towards drugs and the drug culture in general.

The representation of the second bad object aspect is the *rejecting object,* which is characterized by negative feelings. This aspect becomes the *anti-libidinal ego* and represents the negative side of drug use. The effects of the drug wane, the pleasurable feelings end, and the user experiences frustration, helplessness, bitterness, rage and hate. The experience of the bad object representation is similar to Khantzian's (1987) description of the state of dysphoria among drug users, and Blatt's (Blatt, Berman, et al., 1984) findings of pervasive self-criticism in drug addicts.

Patterns of Object Relations Among Drug Users—Fairbairn's Theory

Using Fairbairn's theory of object relations, it is possible to hypothesize that drug addicts regulate their intrapsychic life in the following way. Due to a deficit in early object relations and the internalization of harsh and frustrating parental objects, a person takes drugs which provide a regressive experience of a primary good object. The experience of this primary good object also masks the harsh, introjected (bad) objects and related dysphoric feelings of self-criticism and worthlessness. As the drug wears off, the affect of the bad object representations return all the stronger for being repressed[2]. Nevertheless, the bad objects and the dysphoria they produce are now linked to the drug. If more of the drug can be obtained, the dysphoria can be controlled. The search for the drug recommences and the cycle is complete.

The internalization of bad object representations allows them to be controlled while their influence is repressed. However, since the bad object representations carry tremendous aggressive energy, they threaten to surface and overpower the ego. Fairbairn characterized this as the experience of being 'possessed' (1952). In his writings, Wurmser (1987) also characterizes the drug-using patient as one who is demonically possessed. Drug users report feeling a loss of control when under the influence of a drug. This alternates with a feeling of being in control when the drug wears off. This cycle of control is very important. If the cycle of use and subsequent withdrawal from the drug is not maintained, it becomes difficult for the drug user to maintain control over his internalized bad object representations. This type of problem can be seen among recovering drug addicts. As

---

[2]Fairbairn spoke of the repression of bad object representations which is not to be confused with normal or neurotic repression. Fairbairn's idea of the repression of object representations is more like what would now be called splitting, or denial in the service of splitting.

Blatt, Berman, et al. (1984) and Wurmser (1974) report, drug addicts who abstain from using can become intensely depressed, hostile, rageful and suicidal. The drug has served to keep their bad object representations in check. When the drug is removed, the bad object representations threaten to surface.

The bad internalized object representations are repressed with the assistance of the internalized good object representation (ideal ego). The good internal object representation acts as a conscience, passing judgment on the bad object representations to keep them in check. In the standard Freudian terminology, the internalized good object representation acts as the *superego* (although this superego is archaic). In the compulsive drug user this internalized good object representation produces a state of controlled dysphoria in the drug user. Therefore, treatment which only reinforces the superego (using moralistic or strongly didactic methods of therapy) is not likely to reduce the craving for drugs, but may instead reinforce their use. The superego of the compulsive drug user inhibits the expression of rage derived from the repressed bad object representations. The healthy expression of anger or rage concomitant with the release of the internalized bad object representations is an important step in the resolution of the split between bad and good object representations.

The good object also has an external representation which aids in the release of the internalized bad object representations in healthy individuals. This leads to mature, differentiated relations with external objects, which in Fairbairn's view is the benchmark for normalcy. Drug users have often never had a good external object (parental figure). As has been outlined, drug use compensates for this external good object. This leads the drug user to idealize the properties of a drug. Typically, drug users characterize their drugs as the "best", "rarest", etc. Freud himself demonstrated this idealizing aspect in his writings on cocaine;

> There is, moreover, in this essay a tone that never recurred in Freud's writings, a remarkable warmth as if he were in love with the content itself. He used expressions uncommon in a scientific paper, such as "the most gor-

geous excitement" that animals display after the injection of cocaine, and administering an "offering" of it rather than a "dose"; he heatedly rebuffed the "slander" that had been published about this precious drug. (Jones, 1961, p. 55)

The compensatory nature of a drug is enhanced by its idealization. This idealization can only be accomplished through a separation of good and bad object representations. Bad object representations are internalized to distance them from the external good object representations. This effects a protection of the external good object representation, allowing it to exist in an idealized state. The maintenance of the good object representation in an idealized protected state is especially important when there has been a loss of the actual external object (mother or guardian). As Fairbairn says,

The loss of an object is thus very much more devastating in the case of an infant...He has no alternative but to accept or to reject his object—an alternative which is liable to present itself to him as a choice between life and death. (Fairbairn, 1952, p. 47)

In this case, the split of external good and internal bad object representations serves to preserve the external object representation. It is not surprising, therefore, to find that habitual drug users usually have a history of early object loss (D. Hartmann, 1969), a phenomenon which has been associated with suicide (Blatt, Rounsaville, et al., 1984; Fine, 1972; Khantzian, 1990; Wasserman & Culberg, 1989; Wurmser, 1974).

By internalizing the representation of the bad objects, the lost good aspects of the external object representation are preserved. It has been suggested that drug users have a difficult time internalizing good object representations. A "...'good external object' is either not there to be seen, or it is not strong enough to overcome the negative one. It cannot be safely introjected" (Luzzatto, 1987, p. 26). The use of a drug, therefore, may represent a compensatory attempt to internalize the good object representation by internalizing its substitute. This internalization may be an attempt to introject the good object so it can control the bad object representation and hence the drug user's dysphoria. This attempt, however, backfires and does not lead to the internalization of the good object representation. Instead, for the drug abuser, the pleasurable aspects of the drug are cathected to hostile parental introjects, causing the drug to be incorporated as both bad and good object representations. As outlined above, when the pleasant effects of the drug wear off, so too does the experience of the good object that was incorporated along with the bad. This leaves only the internalized bad object representation. Once again there is only an external good object representation and an internal bad object representation; the split remains. The state of dysphoria continues and the drug abuser will eventually repeat the use of drugs in order to attempt once more to incorporate the good object. Whether or not this leads to pathological problems depends on the extent of the internalization, the degree of badness of the object, the extent to which the ego is identified with the bad object representations, and the nature and strengths of the ego's defenses against the bad object representations.

Object Constancy

Fairbairn's theory of object relations serves as a useful backdrop for understanding patterns of compulsive drug use. Nevertheless, more modern conceptions and theories of object relations can help to delineate these patterns more clearly. One such concept is that of object constancy. Object constancy, according to H. Hartmann (1952) refers to the mental representation of a loved object which remains internally within the mind of the infant, independent of his state of needs. In other words, when the infant reaches a state of object constancy he can maintain the mental representation of the object whether or not he has a need to be satisfied. The constant object representation is an internalized positively cathected mother image. In other words, object constancy represents the presence of a consistent and internalized representation of a good object. Mahler, Pine and Bergman (1975), however, expand the idea of object constancy to represent a consistent object representation which is a fusion of both internalized bad and good object representations.

> ...the constancy of the object implies more than the maintenance of the representation of the absent love object...It also implies the unifying of the "good" and "bad" object into one whole representation. This fosters the fusion of the aggressive and libidinal drives and tempers the hatred for the object when aggression is intense. (p. 110)

The presence of a consistent internalized object representation allows the infant to tolerate frustration, anxiety and aggression which result from the temporary loss of the external good object (mother). Along with Hoffer (1955), Mahler, Bergman and Pine (1975) believe that object constancy should be thought of as "the last stage of a mature object relationship" (p. 110). Drug users attempt to internalize a representation of a good object which is not consistent and, therefore, suffer from profound object relations pathology. The achievement of object constancy is most likely the clearest single differentiating phenomenon between drug users and abusers. Although Blatt, Berman, et al. (1984) have characterized opiate addicts as having a neurotic level of pathology, they have also indicated severe deficits in the capacity of drug addicts to maintain gratifying object relations. Given the hostile, self-critical nature of the parental introjects of addicts and their difficulty controlling affect, it is highly unlikely that they have reached a level of mature object relations.

Patterns of Object Relations Among Drug Users—Modern Theories

When object constancy has not been achieved, good and bad object representations remain split off from one another. In pathological cases of drug use this can mean that good and bad object representations are split off to an even greater degree. To maintain this split, the compulsive drug user will increase his use of drugs. The drug serves to maintain the good object representation by providing affect related to the good object. The compulsive drug user must keep increasing his drug use to maintain the pleasurable affect as he habituates to the drug's effect. Paradoxically, this increase in the use of drugs also maintains the bad object representation by providing more negative affect as the drug wears off. Therefore, drug use can be understood energizing both good and bad object representations. When these object representations have increased energy, it is more difficult to maintain the defensive splitting of the good and bad object representations. Therefore, in order to preserve the good object representation, the bad object representation will be projected, or externalized, with the concomitant release of rage and hostility. In this way, compulsive drug use can be seen as a projection-introjection cycle similar to the dynamic found in borderline personality syndrome (Kernberg, 1967, 1975). The major difference is that the introjective aspect of the cycle is externally controlled through the ingestion of drugs, while the projective aspect of the cycle is internally controlled by a habituation to the drug's effects. This cycle of projection and introjection maintains the split necessary to maintain ego functioning. Nevertheless, due to the physiological nature of drug use, especially the body's habituation to the effects of the drug, this cycle functions in a positive feedback loop. This means that with compulsive drug use, this cycle becomes increasingly difficult to maintain (Of course, this difficulty varies depending upon the drug used). If the split cannot be maintained, the ego may dissociate causing a psychotic break. The compulsive drug user must, therefore, perform a balancing act, constantly monitoring the introjective (ingesting of the drug) and projective (habituation to the drug's effects) sides of the cycle, regulating the libidinal and aggressive drive energy in the object/ego (self) system. This theory would seem to explain why drug users, when seen in extreme states, alternate between states of violent agitation and profound emotional withdrawal. Interestingly enough, it is possible that those who are considered to be the most pathological drug users, i.e. opiate addicts, can best perform this balancing act. A study by McLellan, Woody and O'Brien (1979) found that users of stimulants over a period of six years showed significant increases in psychotic level pathology (including mania, paranoia and schizophrenia). Users of depressants over the same period showed an increase in general pathology, non-psychotic depression and cognitive impairment. Contrary to intuition, opiate addicts showed no change in level of pathology during the same period, except for some mild increase in depression. There was no evidence of psychotic or organic impairment among the opiate addicts.

Eventually, the ego may try and destroy the bad object representations. Unfortunately, this can lead to the literal destruction of the individual, in which the battle is won at the cost of losing the war. This may be a possible explanation for the phenomenon of apparent and non-apparent (overdoses, accidental deaths, etc.) suicides among habitual drug users.

Drugs as Transitional Objects

The significance of the object relations dynamics outlined above, can also be understood through Winnicott's concept of the transitional object (Winnicott, 1951; 1989). Winnicott, contrary to other psychoanalysts of the British School, conceptualized object relations as an infant's relationship with its primary caretakers, especially the relationship to the mother. For other analysts, objects tend to be thought of as fantasies or projections of the infant which result from drive satisfaction. Fairbairn, a contemporary of Winnicott, postulated that these objects carried their own energy and thus freed object relations from Freudian drive theory. Winnicott very much admired the relational aspects of Fairbairn's theories of object relations and Winnicott's work can be seen as bridging the gap between the drive and relational theories of object relations.

Winnicott saw object relationships as developing from infantile fantasy or projection, but ending up as concrete human interaction, most often between a mother and her baby. Infantile fantasy and projection play important roles in object relations, but the role is to aid in the establishment of actual relationships. Winnicott's transitional object is crucial in this regard. For the infant, early development proceeds from a state of omnipotence and control over the universe to an eventual understanding that there are events and phenomena outside his sphere of control. Transitional objects bridge this developmental period and are crucial to its successful navigation.

Transitional objects are things that are familiar to the infant, such as a blanket, thumb or fingers, the mother's breast or other parts of her body, etc. The infant projects or endows these real objects with drive tension reducing qualities. The drive tension reduction of the transitional object then begins to coincide with the administering of the actual mother or caretaker. Eventually, under the modulation of the mother or caretaker, the transitional object is understood by the infant to be a separate entity. As Winnicott says,

> At first whatever object gains a relationship with the infant is created by the infant...It is like a hallucination. Some cheating takes place and an object that is ready to hand overlaps with an hallucination. Obviously the way the mother or her substitute behaves is of paramount importance here. One mother is good and another bad at letting a real object be just where the infant is hallucinating an object so that in fact the infant gains the illusion that the world can be created and what is created is the world. (Winnicott, 1989, p. 53)

After a transitional object can be experienced by the infant as existing as a separate entity, this separateness is soon extended to other objects. The infant begins to relate to the world as being outside himself. The external objects in the world can now also take on symbolic value for the infant. In normal development, the transitional object is soon left behind as the infant develops an interest in the world around him. However, in times of distress, or if the transition is not modulated correctly by the mother, a clinging (or in older individuals, a regression) to transitional objects can occur. An infant will become very disturbed if a transitional object is removed. If the transitional object is lost, the infant will replace it with a similar object after a period of withdrawal (Greenacre, 1969).

It is quite likely that if the primary object (mother) is not available to the infant, or to use Winnicott's terminology, she is not a "good enough" mother, the infant is unable to distinguish between the primary object and an inanimate transitional object. As D. Rosenfeld says,

> The physical relation, the skin-to-skin contact with their mother is so disturbed, so vitiated, so spurious and bizarre, that the patient is indifferent to whether he is with a warm-skinned mother or with an inanimate life-less object. (1992, p. 238)

This analogy can be extended to compulsive drug users, who cannot distinguish between the experience of the primary object and the experience of the drug. For these individuals, drugs are like inanimate transitional objects, or more accurately, the *reactivated* transitional objects described by V. Volkan (1981). These reactivated transitional objects serve to defend against object relations conflicts rather than working towards their resolution. In other words, the experience of the transitional object in later childhood or adult life is associated with a change in their original function. Originally, transitional objects served to promote healthy growth. When used in later childhood or adulthood, however, the function of the now reactivated transitional object is to maintain a state of psychopathology. V. Volkan (1981, 1988) suggests that there are a number of different types of magical objects (all connected to the original transitional objects) that serve to maintain pathology. These include, *the childhood fetish, the childhood psychotic fetish, suitable targets for externalization, the classical fetish, substitute objects, linking objects, phobic objects* and *keepsakes, talismans,* or *ornaments.* The following is a brief description of each:

1. *The childhood fetish* is an object which functions as a pathological defense against preoedipal separation from the mother. In this type of fetish, the object replaces the gratifying aspects of the mother (e.g. the breast).

2. *The childhood psychotic fetish* is an object which is used
   in a bizarre way when the child breaks with reality.
   The child uses the object to repair a psychotic perception of body defect which stems from an incomplete
   separation from the mother.

3. *A suitable target for externalization* is an object which
   absorbs the child's unmended self and object images.
   These images serve to stabilize the self and object representations of the children and help them bond more
   closely with the group. These object images often take
   the form of cultural amplifiers such as flags or ethnic
   costumes and are shared among children in an ethnic
   or racial group.

4. *The classical fetish* is related to castration anxiety and is
   usually employed by a male to represent an imagined
   mother's penis.

5. *Substitute objects* are used by adult schizophrenics in
   the same way that children use the psychotic fetish.

6. *Phobic objects* become symbols for areas of conflict to
   be avoided.

7. *Linking objects* connect the mourner to a representation of a lost object. Linking objects range from being
   bizarre to being aesthetically pleasing.

8. *Keepsakes, talismans, or ornaments* are objects that are
   used to defend against separation and castration
   anxiety. These objects are usually invested with magical power and have cultural significance with multiple layers of meaning.

What distinguishes these reactivated transitional objects
from one another are the psychodynamic processes involved
in each. Drugs are probably most like childhood psychotic
fetishes or substitute objects, as they are incorporated to protect the compulsive drug user's reality testing (by maintain-

ing the split between good and bad object representations). Drugs also provide enhanced self-esteem through the experience of pleasurable affect and a sense of control over dysphoria by the user. In this way, drugs also come to have magical properties for the user.

The above view, however, does not preclude drugs, as inanimate objects, from representing the other types of reactivated transitional objects listed above. Most of the object types listed above are related to some difficulty in early infant - mother interaction. The use of drugs as reactivated transitional objects is reminiscent of both the pleasurable and the frustrating aspects of the mother. For instance, Berman (Berman, 1972; V. Volkan, 1976) has documented a case of a young women who compulsively used amphetamines in pill form. Although he originally saw the drug as a fetish, he came to realize that it functioned as a reactivated transitional object. The amphetamine pills were seen as a representation of food. The amphetamines also gave the patient a sense of well-being and warmth which was closely associated with a transitional object. Also (in diet pill form), the amphetamines prevented eating. Therefore, the amphetamines symbolized both the good nourishing and the bad depriving mother. Drug use attempts to recreate the pleasurable aspects of the mother via the transitional object, while defending against her frustrating and anxiety provoking deficits.

The use of drugs as a reactivated transitional object has other negative ramifications. For the normal infant the transitional object phase is important in that the ability to symbolize affective and perceptual phenomena has its genesis during this time. If the infant is not able to successfully negotiate the transitional object stage and instead uses objects pathologically (like a fetish), his ability to symbolize and express affect will be compromised. For such individuals, affect cannot be symbolized into language and expressed. Instead it is acted out in a compulsive and impulsive fashion (Krystal, 1977). This is reminiscent of McDougall's (1984) description of disaffected patients who,

> ...were unable to contain or cope with phases of highly charged affectivity (precipitated as often as not by external events). They saw no choice but to plunge into some

form of action to dispel the threatened upsurge of emotion. It might be emphasized that this could apply to exciting and agreeable affects as well as to painful ones. (p.
389)

Defects in the transitional object phase of infancy could be an
explanation for the impulsivity, compulsivity and abnormal
affect seen in drug users. As has been previously noted,
these defects are often triggered by the real or imagined loss
of a primary object in infancy. If the primary object or caretaker was not lost, then this person (mother or the father) often presented conflicting messages to her child. McDougall
(1985), in her writings on what she calls the *normopath*, describes the typical object relations pattern of the compulsive
drug user,

> In several personal histories among both the acting-out
> and the normopathic patients, one parent, usually the fa-
> ther, had died or left the family in the patient's early in-
> fancy. The mothers were frequently presented as over-
> possessive and overattentive while at the same time
> heedless of the child's affective states. In other instances
> the mother seemed to have been psychologically absent
> because of depression or psychotic episodes. These
> mothers appeared to have been too close or too distant in
> their relationship to their babies. It seemed to me that,
> for whatever reasons, a truly caretaking mother-image
> had never been introjected into the child's inner psychic
> structure, there to remain as an object of identification,
> allowing the child to become a good parent to itself.
> Thus in adult life the original maternal image, essential
> for dealing with emotional as well as physical pain and
> states of overstimulation, continued to be sought un-
> remittingly in the external world in the form of addictive
> substances...I have referred to these activities as patho-
> logical transitional or transitory objects. (p. 157)

In this sense, drugs also function as what V. Volkan
(1981) terms linking objects. These are a variety of transitional objects which are more highly symbolic of the loss of
the primary object or caretaker. In general, reactivated transitional objects recreate the pleasurable aspects of the mother
while attempting to defend against her deficits. Linking objects, being related to the loss of the object, may compensate
the mother's loss first and defend against her deficits second.
When the drug experience is weighted more heavily on tak-

ing the mother's place, then the drug is more like a linking object. It can be hypothesized that some drugs, like opiates, function more like linking object because they produce experiences related more closely to the pleasurable aspects of the mother. These feelings, consciously or unconsciously, serve to 'link' the user to a lost object to which he has had an ambivalent relationship. Many other drugs produce an intrapsychic state which is not as directly pleasurable and are perhaps more related to psychic defenses like splitting. Drugs, such as LSD, often induce paradoxical feelings of intense separateness and relatedness which are not always pleasurable. These drugs, when used compulsively (remember they are not addictive), therefore, function more like a psychotic fetish, in that they attempt to repair a perception of an incomplete self or body image. It is not surprising to find that this class of drugs was thought for a long time to be psychomimetic.

Summary and Conclusions

In this chapter I have outlined the basic tenets of developmental object relations theory and how it is manifested in drug use pathology. The phenomenology of compulsive drug users indicates that their object relations dynamics have aspects of the dynamics of good and bad object representations as described by Fairbairn (1952). In a more modern sense, Kernberg's (1967, 1975) conceptualization of borderline pathology, shows that the drug user is unable to integrate good and bad object representations. Instead drugs are used in an attempt to maintain the defensive splitting between good and bad object representations. This type of compulsive drug use also serves to energize a cycle of introjection and projection of object representations. Seen in light of modern object relations theories, drugs serve as transitional objects, which reactivate a link to the good and bad aspects of the primary object. For most compulsive drug users, the transitional stage of object relations is not resolved. This has important ramifications for the treatment of drug use pathology. These ramifications are most important in the clinical setting, requiring the psychotherapist to function in the role of the transitional object, while eventually moving the drug using patient's dependence on drugs to a more healthy state.

Chapter Five

From Mythology to Case History

In this chapter, theoretical formulations about the role of drugs in the psychic life of the individual will be demonstrated through the presentation of a number of cases. The case study methodology has historically been the method of choice for psychoanalytic-oriented studies. Although the case study method has come under criticism from both psychoanalytic and non-psychoanalytic sources, it is my opinion that it is still the most valid and appropriate method for describing material related to the intrapsychic life of the individual. Because of the importance of the case study it will be useful to examine the different uses of this methodology within the psychoanalytic literature. (For a more encompassing discussion of case study methodology and related issues see Cambell & Stanley, 1963; Fisher & Greenberg, 1985; Giorgi, 1970; Runyan, 1980; Sarnoff, 1971; Romanyshyn, 1978; Trepper, 1990; K. Volkan, 1993).

The Use of The Case Study Method in Psychoanalytic Research

Within the strict framework of psychoanalytic theory there is much support for the use of case studies. Freud (1933) clearly understood the advantages of the case study method, while recognizing that it was not a scholarly panacea.

> Its therapeutic successes give grounds neither for boast-
> ing nor for being ashamed. But statistics...are in general
> misinstructive; the material worked upon is so heteroge-
> neous that only very large numbers would show any-
> thing. It is wiser to examine one's individual experi-
> ences. (p. 152)

Since Freud, other writers have extolled the virtues of the
case study method. For instance, Meadow (1984), understands the case study to be an integral part of the psychoanalytic method. Analytic writers like Edelson (1988) and Langs
(1976) believe that the subjective experience of the analyst is
of the utmost importance and that this should be included in
the scientific understanding of clinical phenomena. This is
especially true when the analyst or psychotherapist is report-
ing on issues related to transference and countertransference
phenomena (Boyer, 1979a, 1983, 1992; Boyer & Giovacchini,
1990, 1992; Giovacchini, 1989). This psychoanalytic understanding of scientific research is similar to the practice of
ethnographic (Borg & Gall, 1983) and phenomenological
(Valle & King, 1978) research. Indeed, these similarities in
scientific understanding may explain the recent cross-fertil-
ization between anthropology and psychoanalysis (Boyer,
1978, 1979b, 1983, Boyer, Boyer, Dithrich, Harned, Hippler,
Stone, & Walt, 1989; Ciambelli & Portanova, 1980; DeVos &
Boyer, 1989; Rabow, 1983). Lagache (1966) relying primarily
upon evidence gathered through case studies argues that
psychoanalysis is an exact science, at least in the production
of an understanding of unconscious processes. This understanding of psychoanalysis is also similar to an ethnographic
and phenomenological understanding of science.

Although there is much general agreement about the usefulness of case material for psychoanalytic study, there is
some disagreement on what case material should be used.
French analyst, Green (1986) has argued that the presentation of one's own cases is not desirable. He believes that
publishing one's own case histories does a disservice to the
patient. Green believes that case studies do not constitute
proof of a specific theory because clinical material can be
presented in such a way as to support almost any theory.
Therefore, it is not worth the possibility of upsetting one's

patients to publish their case histories. This criticism, however, does not apply to previously published case histories and some psychoanalytic researchers believe it is more appropriate to conduct a secondary analysis of case examples from the literature than to present one's own cases (Trevisano, 1990).

In addition to the use of previously published clinical material, non-clinical case histories have increasingly been the subject of psychoanalytic investigation. This material has consisted primarily of mythological, historical, and biographical case histories. The analysis of these types of case histories falls within the parameters of the case study method as it has been generally defined in the social sciences (Borg & Gall, 1983). Each type of case history is discussed briefly below.

Mythological Case Studies

Mythology has been studied in psychoanalysis since Freud first elucidated the importance of the Oedipus myth for the understanding of human psychology. The relevance of mythology for psychoanalysis today is clearly demonstrated in a paper by Pollock (1986) who suggests that the Oedipus myth and its subsequent representations in literature present a complete picture of human conflicts and intrapsychic dynamics. Other psychoanalytic studies of mythology include analyses of the hero myth (Rosenman, 1988), rites of passage (Gayda & Vacola, 1988), religious mythology (Almansi, 1983) and the myth of Dionysus (Dubosc-Benabou, 1990). Overall, mythological studies are a cornerstone and a unique feature of psychoanalytic science and inquiry.

Psychohistory and Psychobiography

The psychoanalytic study of historical data has led to the creation of the field of psychohistory. This type of inquiry seeks to understand past events through the psychodynamic motivation of important historical figures and populations of individuals. In other words, psychohistory seeks to psycho-analytically understand why people acted in a certain way in the past (Lawton, 1990). Examples of psychohistorical studies include Kestenberg & Brenner's (1985) study of children who survived the holocaust, Lifton's (1968) study of Mao Tse-tung and Chinese politics, and V. Volkan's study of conflict in the Mideast (V. Volkan, 1979; V. Volkan & Itzkowitz, 1984).

Obviously, psychohistory is related to psychobiography, or the study of significant individuals who lived in the past. Psychobiographical studies may or may not be related to historical events. Indeed, many historically significant individuals have been studied for their interesting clinical characteristics as well as their historical significance. Freud's (1910, 1939) work on Leonardo da Vinci and Moses were the first psychoanalytic psychobiographies. More recent psychoanalytic psychobiographical studies include the lives of William Faulkner (Martin, 1983), Jimi Hendrix (K. Volkan, 1991), Catherine de Medici (Adams-Silvan & Adams, 1986), Marilyn Monroe (Chessick, 1982), Bertrand Russell (Brink, 1985), George Sand (Deutsch, 1982), and Virginia Woolf (Panken, 1983).

Psychopathy and the Psychobiography of the Artist

It is not surprising that many psychobiographical subjects are artists, musicians or writers. According to Kris (1952) the inspiration to produce a work of art has psychodynamic underpinnings. Therefore, the study of those individuals who have left a legacy of creative work is likely to lead to a richer understanding of their intrapsychic life. Freud (1910) coined the term *pathography* to describe the psychoanalytic study of the creative work of these individuals. Recently, Spitz (1985, 1987, 1991) has brilliantly applied the use of psychobiography and pathography to study the relation of object dynamics to artistic expression in a number of artists and musicians. For Spitz it is important for the researcher to try and reconstruct the early childhood experiences and fantasies, early object relations, drive & drive derivatives with regard to psychosexual stages, and oedipal conflicts which occur in the life of the artist. One of the difficulties of constructing a psychobiography is obtaining information on the early life of the subject. When this information is sketchy, an examination of the art of the subject can be invaluable in supporting psychodynamic hypotheses about his or her early life.

In summary, it would appear that the positive outcomes of the case study method far outweigh the negative outcomes. While the case study method does not adhere to a strict scientific paradigm, other frameworks such as the judicial paradigm allow for the rigorous testing of competing hypotheses which arise from the interpretation of case material (K. Volkan, 1993). The case study method excels at providing rich levels of detail necessary for the construction of *grounded* theories which account for the subjective bias of the researcher. This is especially relevant for psychoanalytic-oriented studies in which the subjective experience of the analyst is essential to the understanding of the phenomena presented by the case material.

Case studies have a wide variety of methodologies, including the analysis of clinical, mythological, historical, and psychobiographical cases. All of these types of case studies are generally acceptable within the social sciences and have been widely applied in psychoanalytic research. Within psychoanalytic research, there is increasing support for the secondary analysis of clinical material and the interpretation of non-clinical material from biographical, historical and mythological sources.

The Myth of Dionysus

With regards to drug use the most prevalent myth from Western sources is the Greek myth of Dionysus (or Bacchus in Latin), the god of wine. The myth of Dionysus elucidates many of the object relations dynamics covered so far in this text. The material on Dionysus used here is largely taken from Euripides (1954), Hamilton (1940) and Kerényi (1951).

Dionysus was born in Thebes, the son of Zeus and the mortal woman Semele. Zeus was in love with Semele and offered to grant her any wish she desired. Unfortunately, she asked Zeus to appear to her in his naked heavenly splendor as the Lord of the Thunderbolt. This idea was, of course, given to Semele by Hera, Zeus' jealous wife. Although Zeus was reluctant to fulfill this wish, Semele reminded him that he had taken an oath on the sacred river Styx. Zeus therefore appeared to Semele in his burning glory, killing her. Before Semele died, Zeus snatched her yet unborn child and ensconced him in his hip to hide him from Hera,

> And the pains of child-birth bound his mother fast,
> And she cast him forth untimely,
> And under the lightning's lash relinquished life;
> And Zeus the son of Cronos
> Ensconced him instantly in a secret womb
> Chambered within his thigh,
> And with golden pins closed him from Hera's sight.
> (Euripides, 1954, p. 194)

When it was time for him to be born, Zeus took Dionysus from his hip and gave him to the Nymphs of Nysa to be raised. When Dionysus reached manhood he wandered over the earth and was accepted everywhere as a god, except in his native land of Greece.

While on his way to Greece, Dionysus was captured and held for ransom by a group of pirates who thought him the son of a king. Ignoring signs of his divinity, the pirates tried to take him away on board their ship. At first Dionysus was passive, even friendly toward the pirates, who with the exception of the helmsman, refused to see the significance of their inability to bind Dionysus with rope. As soon as he was bound, the ropes came undone. Eventually, wine began to run in streams down the deck and vines grew upon the mast. Dionysus turned into a roaring lion and all the sailors, except the helmsman jumped into the sea and were turned into dolphins.

Dionysus missed his lost mother terribly and finally decided to retrieve her from the underworld. As Hamilton (1940) says,

The mother he had never seen was not forgotten. He longed for her so greatly that at last he dared the terrible descent to the lower world to seek her...Dionysus brought her away, but not to live on earth. He took her up to Olympus, where the gods consented to receive her as one of themselves...(p. 56)

Dionysus was also known for his worshippers, the Maenads (or Bacchantes). These were women who lived in the wilderness upon herbs, berries and goat's milk. The Maenads would become frenzied with wine drinking and rush through the woods until they came upon a living creature. At this point they would literally rip, bite and tear the creature to pieces, devouring the bloody flesh. The Maenads, who were commonly thought to be madwomen (our word 'mania' originated from 'Maenad'; cf. Kerényi, 1951), lived in a world both beautiful and ecstatic as well as degrading and brutal. As Hamilton (1940) says,

They woke to a sense of peace and heavenly freshness; they bathed in a clear brook. There was much that was lovely, good and freeing in their worship under the open sky and the ecstasy of joy it brought in the wild beauty of the world. And yet always present, too, was the horrible bloody feast. (p. 57).

Perhaps the best-known story of Dionysus is his encounter with his cousin Pentheus, King of Thebes. This story is the basis of Euripides' tragedy, *The Bacchae* (1954). When Thebes is beset with crazed Maenads, Pentheus orders them imprisoned along with their leader. Although Pentheus is warned by his elder advisors that this leader is Dionysus, a god, he refuses to believe them. Dionysus does not put up any resistance to arrest and is brought to Pentheus. At first he is timid and meek. Once again, fetters fail to hold Dionysus as well as the Maenads, who escape into the hills to drink wine and hold wild sexual orgies. Much to Pentheus' dismay the Maenads take many Thebian women with them, including his mother and sister. Pentheus is very angry with Dionysus who remains calm and gentle, although he warns Pentheus that,

...."god will set me free",
"God?", Pentheus asks jeeringly.
"Yes", Dionysus answered. "He is here and sees my suf-
fering".
"Not where my eyes can see him", Pentheus said.
"He is here where I am", answered Dionysus.
"You cannot see him because you are not pure".
(Hamilton, 1940, p. 58)

Eventually, Dionysus escapes and Pentheus sets out to
retrieve the Thebian women, including his mother and sister,
from the Maenads' frenzied carousing. Dionysus makes all
the women mad and they rush upon Pentheus, tearing him
from limb-to-limb,

A single and continuous yell arose—Pentheus
Shrieking as long as life was left in him, the women
Howling in triumph. One of them carried off an arm,
Another a foot, the boot still laced on it. The ribs
Were stripped, clawed clean; and the women's hands,
thick red with blood,
Were tossing, catching, like a plaything, Pentheus'
flesh...
His poor head—His mother carries it, fixed on her thyr-
sus-point...
She has left her sisters
Dancing among the Maenads...
Inside the walls, exulting in her hideous prey,
Shouting to Bacchus, calling him her fellow-hunter...
(Euripides, 1954, pp. 233-234)

When their senses return, the women realize that Pentheus
has been their bloody feast.

The myth of Dionysus is illustrative of many of the intrapsychic dynamics seen in compulsive drug users. To begin with there is the early loss of the primary object. It seems
that Dionysus is the only god whose mother was mortal.
Therefore, much of his mythology is devoted to proving and
maintaining his narcissistic sense of omnipotence. The combination of a weak (i.e. mortal) mother and an overbearing
omnipotent father seem to be the cause of the basic flaw in
Dionysus' psychic make-up. Semele is impulsive and this
combined with the suggestion of the jealous Hera results in
her destruction by an all-powerful father/lover. The omnipotent father-figure destroys the mother and then completely envelops the embryonic Dionysus, taking on the

mothering role. This is the same dynamic seen in the cases of the five amphetamine addicted women described later in the chapter, in which the father also takes on the early mothering role. In these cases, as in the myth of Dionysus, it is also the father's narcissism which destroys the mother and disables her ability to take care of her children. The fathers then subsequently abandoned their offspring. This is also true in the myth of Dionysus. For soon after Dionysus is born, he is abandoned by his father.

When Dionysus' omnipotent narcissism is questioned, as in his encounter with the pirates, he first responds with a seemingly calm sense of detachment. After a time, however, this calm defense gives way to a primitive oral rage (in the pirate story, Dionysus becomes a roaring lion) which serves to maintain Dionysus' sense of divine omnipotence. Dionysus is able to maintain this sense of omnipotence everywhere except in his land of origin. In psychological terms, Dionysus is the perfect narcissist until he can no longer use this as a defense against his object relations defects. Dionysus attempts to repair these defects by retrieving the representation of the lost good object. Although Dionysus is able to retrieve this good mother object from the land of the dead, she must be idealized and protected by placement in Olympus among the gods. This idealization of the good object representation is reminiscent of the splitting of good and bad object representations. The splitting off of the good object representation (the idealized mother in Olympus) coincides with the denial of the bad object representation. In this case the bad object representation takes on a number of forms. It can be seen as the dangerous all-powerful father, Zeus, who is hardly mentioned later in the myth of Dionysus, or as Dionysus' rage which surfaces from time to time. Other sections of the myth of Dionysus clearly show this split between good and bad object representations as well. For instance Dionysus' followers, the Maenads are either pure and clean, living a holy existence in the wilderness, or they are degenerate murderers and cannibals enjoying the bloody fruits of their oral aggression. It is also of interest to recall that it is the wine itself which catalyzes these split qualities in the Maenads. The fetters which are unable to bind Dionysus and his followers may point to the inability of the compulsive drug user to integrate, or bind, the split object representations into a cohesive self.

The story of Pentheus is a tale of the retribution of the bad object representations. Pentheus refuses to help Dionysus maintain his omnipotent narcissistic defenses against integration. As seen in the above quotation, Pentheus refuses to recognize Dionysus' divinity and insists that Dionysus submit to imprisonment. In other words, Pentheus represents an attempt to integrate the object representations. The result is that Dionysus must flee. The bad object representation, fueled by oral aggression, rises up and 'possesses' the Maenads who destroy the ego (Pentheus) in a bloody feast.

The myth of Dionysus describes many of the dynamics of the compulsive drug user. The loss of the early objects, the narcissistic father, the split of bad and good object representation, the violent return of the bad object representation, oral aggression and rage, and pathological narcissism are all reminiscent of the compulsive drug user, especially in the sense of the borderline drug addict described by Kernberg (1975). In the myth of Dionysus, the wine, like drugs of all types, helps to maintain these pathological object relation dynamics.

Thomas DeQuincy and the Confessions of an Opium Eater

The next case is another historical example, this time of an opiate addict. This case will illustrate many of the dynamics reported by recent psychoanalytic writers.

Thomas DeQuincy was an English intellectual and writer of the 19th century. He is largely known for his *Confessions of an English Opium Eater*, although he produced numerous lesser works (DeQuincy, 1985). DeQuincy was an opium addict for much of his life, though he fought his addiction and during a few periods achieved abstinence from the drug. His life history has been excellently chronicled by Ward (1966).

Thomas DeQuincy was born in 1785 to a large family that was moderately well-off financially. His father was a merchant and his mother the daughter of a military officer. DeQuincy's mother was an efficient parent, but probably not very affectionate. His father seems to have spent a good deal of time traveling on business. Young Thomas was the favorite of his sisters who doted on him during his infancy. Unfortunately, DeQuincy's early childhood was tainted by a series of losses. In quick succession his grandmother and younger sister Jane died when he was five. Two years later, his best loved sister, Elizabeth died, leaving DeQuincy profoundly affected. After Elizabeth's death, DeQuincy became increasingly isolated and buried himself in intellectual pursuits. One year later, his father, who had spent much time away from home, returned so that he could die at home of tuberculosis. DeQuincy experienced profound guilt over the death of his father, which he could not understand. As a result of his father's death, DeQuincy's older brother William returned to the family from boarding school. William despised his younger brother and spent much effort to humiliate and torment him. Besides his brother, DeQuincy was left in the charge of different tutors and guardians. In school, DeQuincy' work was brilliant, especially in the classics. Nevertheless, he was much bullied by his schoolmates. By the time he was 15, DeQuincy wished to enter Oxford. Nevertheless, his mother insisted that he continue at grammar school. After a period of unsuccessful rebellion, DeQuincy ran away from school for a period of four months. During this time he lived in destitute poverty and his only friend was a young prostitute named Ann. Eventually, DeQuincy returned home and soon after he enrolled at Oxford. In college DeQuincy continued to live without friends or much human contact, preferring instead to immerse himself in his studies. It was during his years at college that he began to use opium. DeQuincy did make two important friends in college, however; Coleridge and Wordsworth. Coleridge was also to become famous for his use of opium along with his literary talents (For a psychoanalytic treatment of Coleridge and his work see Mahon, 1987). DeQuincy's relationship to Wordsworth was to practically become a member of his family. He lived in close proximity and when Wordsworth's young daughter died, DeQuincy was completely undone. He began to take opium daily and his addiction helped to estrange him from Wordsworth. Soon after DeQuincy married and for awhile all seemed to be going well. Predictably, however, DeQuincy's addiction began to consume him. Throughout the next three years, supported by his wife, DeQuincy began to get better and to write. In 1821 he published the *Confessions* which was quite successful. The success of this work enhanced DeQuincy's reputation so that he was able to live off his literary talents. Nevertheless, DeQuincy was plagued by money problems for the rest of his life. He did not produce any other significant work, but instead published numerous small, undistinguished pieces. The *Confessions* remained DeQuincy's magnum opus and he continued to rewrite it throughout his life. After his wife died, DeQuincy was cared for by his six children, most notable his eldest and youngest daughters. Eventually, his health was spent and he died in 1859 at the age of 74.

The impact of DeQuincy's childhood upon his subsequent opium addiction was profound. DeQuincy himself realized this and put much of the blame for his later troubles upon his childhood. In *Suspiria De Profundis* (DeQuincy, 1985), the sequel to the *Confessions*, DeQuincy poses a question from a hypothetical reader,

> "But how came you to take opium in this excess?" The answer to *that* would be: "Because some early events in my life had left a weakness in one organ which required (or seemed to require) that stimulant". (p. 115)

DeQuincy goes on to report on the state of his childhood,

> The particular case to which I refer in my own childhood was one of intolerable grief, a trial, in fact, more severe than many people at *any* age are called upon to stand. (p. 118)

From an account of DeQuincy's life we can assume that his earliest caretakers were his young sisters, who provided DeQuincy with consistent and gratifying primary objects.

The loss of his sisters must have been felt all too keenly. When his younger sister died, DeQuincy felt a sense of awe, but did not experience the loss in a profoundly negative manner. Instead it was the loss of his older sister which quite possibly changed the course of his life. This sister, no doubt took on most of the mothering functions for DeQuincy. His response to this loss was to become withdrawn and isolated in intellectual pursuits. The respite derived from this withdrawal was short-lived as DeQuincy also had to deal with his father's death. DeQuincy's unexplainable guilt over his father's death was no doubt due to an unresolved Oedipus complex. After his father's death, however, DeQuincy was to have no father figure with whom to identify, except his cruel older brother. Although, DeQuincy did not identify with this brother, he no doubt internalized his brother's long-term cruel and demeaning treatment as hostile, negative, self-critical, and harsh introjects, or bad object representations. In DeQuincy's later writings it is readily apparent that these intensely self-critical introjects are functioning. For instance, in the *Confessions* (DeQuincy, 1985) describes his addiction to opium as follows,

> He lies under the weight of incubus and nightmare; he lies in sight of all that he would fain perform, just as a man forcibly confined to bed by the mortal languor of a relaxing disease, who is compelled to witness injury or outrage offered to some object of his tenderest love: he curses the spells which chain him down from motion; he would lay down his life if he might but get up and walk; but he is powerless as an infant and cannot even attempt to rise. (p. 89)

From this quote, the paralyzing power of the bad object representations becomes clear. It is interesting to note that when external events or trauma made greater demands upon DeQuincy, he would increase his dosage of opium until he was incapacitated. Anything in his life that approximated the original loss of the good object (i.e. the death of his elder sister) would cause DeQuincy to compensate by attempting to incorporate the experience of the good object through the effects of opium. For instance, Wordsworth's daughter no doubt reminded DeQuincy of his own sister and he grew very fond and attached to her. When she died, DeQuincy went on an opium binge that was to last for years.

DeQuincy's addiction demonstrates many of the ideas of Blatt, Fairbairn and Khantzian. DeQuincy clearly used opium to effect control over his persuasive feelings of dysphoria. It can be conjectured that he was unable to tolerate the rage and hostility which he must have felt and the drug must have served to keep these feelings in check. Much like many compulsive drug users, DeQuincy also suffered from object loss. Yet because this loss occurred at a later age, DeQuincy was able to stabilize his intrapsychic world to a greater degree than many more primitive drug addicts. Nevertheless, it can be conjectured that a similar dynamic with regard to the good and bad object representations was established. The loss of the good object was compensated for by the drug which was internalized. Once internalized, the good representations of the drug wore off, leaving only the bad, which were then added to DeQuincy's harsh, self-critical introjects. Although severely troubled, it would be a mistake to label DeQuincy as psychotic. His pathology would seem to follow Blatt's assertion that addicts suffer from introjective depression. DeQuincy, over the course of his life, also did not seem to decompensate into a more primitive level of pathology, but more or less, maintained a steady state.

The Case of Jimi Hendrix

Jimi Hendrix was a musician who become famous in the 1960s. Besides his fame as a guitarist, he was also know for his voracious appetite for sex and drugs. From Hendrix' biographies (Henderson, 1981; McDermott, 1992; Shapiro & Glebbeek, 1990) there is a clear picture of his early life as well as his later career as a musician.

Hendrix was abandoned by his mother soon after his birth, as she did not want to be bothered with raising a child. His mother had recurring bouts of tuberculosis. This required her to be immediately separated from her son after birth. When she recovered she showed little interest in the child, preferring instead to stay out all night, drinking and dancing. This served to keep her in precarious health for the remainder of her life. Hendrix' mother divorced her husband during this time while he was away at war. The boy lived with different relatives during much of his early life until his father returned from military service and reclaimed him.

From all accounts Hendrix' father was kind but somewhat withdrawn. He did, however, tend to become stern and authoritative when approached on an affective level. He refused to talk about his feelings and kept them to himself. Young Hendrix suffered greatly from the loss of his mother, although he would see her from time to time. At one point, Hendrix' parents were reunited. This reunion, however, was short-lived. Whenever the young Hendrix asked about his mother, his father would become very authoritative and give him work to do. Although Hendrix' father could not share his feelings with his son he did encourage him to learn the guitar. Hendrix soon became obsessed with the instrument, spending much time alone practicing. Hendrix' mother died when he was eighteen.

Hendrix apparently began using drugs during his high school years. During this time he attended classes but was not a good student. Instead he played in a number of bands which worked regularly. He eventually joined the Air Force (no doubt as an attempt to identify with the father), where he served as a paratrooper. It was during this time that Hendrix displayed noticeably bizarre behavior which alternated between acting out (usually with his guitar), and severe withdrawal. He became something of an outcast and left the service. For the next few years Hendrix worked as a rhythm and blues musician, ending up in Greenwich Village. Hendrix continued to use drugs during this period, primarily amphetamines and marijuana. Hendrix had an unusual habit of storing his supply of amphetamines which was perhaps related to his early object loss.

> Smoking dope to keep mellow and snorting methedrine to keep going was as natural as breathing...Jimmy kept his speed crystals in a baby's bottle, always a source of great amusement. (Shapiro & Glebbeek, 1990, p. 104)

After a number of years of working with different groups, Hendrix formed his own musical style. He was eventually discovered and taken to England to form his band, *The Experience*. Hendrix was heavily swept up in the drug scene of the 1960s. His routine was to use drugs to support a superhuman playing schedule. Hendrix' drug use served to keep him going so that he could play the guitar. Hendrix often reported feeling as if he were possessed, a sentiment he often expressed in his music.

In 1970, while on tour in Germany, Hendrix stayed at the house of a girlfriend. He ate dinner, took some sleeping pills and went to sleep. He never awoke, having asphyxiated on his on vomit. His death has been attributed to factors which include suicide, careless paramedics, or that he did not know the dosage on the brand of sleeping pills he took.

Hendrix' life clearly illustrates aspects of both drive/structure and relational theories of object relations with regard to drug use. He undoubtedly suffered from the loss of his primary object (mother). Passed from relative to relative, Hendrix was never able to attain object constancy (Mahler, Pine & Bergman, 1975). His relationship to his father did not compensate for the loss of his mother. Although his father provided Hendrix with some stability, he was not present on an affective level (cf. Wurmser, 1978). According to Lacan (1982), the "law of the father" was not established. Although Hendrix' father provided some anchoring, he was not entirely stable. As Mitchell (1982) says, "..the father stands in the position...that <u>must</u> break the asocial dyadic unit of mother and child. (p. 28)"

In Hendrix' case, the mother was not available, and the guitar became her substitute. Hendrix's father did not break the dyad between Hendrix and his guitar, but instead encouraged it. It is not surprising that Hendrix became a great guitarist. It is also not surprising that he exhibited many schizoid tendencies, alternating between withdrawal and acting out. Nevertheless, Hendrix' father was not harsh, punitive, and physically or emotionally abusive. If this had been the case it is possible that Hendrix' pathology would have increased to the point where he would have become an addict (cf. Blatt, Rounsaville, et al., 1984).

For Hendrix, the guitar became a compensatory object, to be protected, preserved and most importantly, played. Hendrix idealized the guitar through playing it. For Hendrix, the guitar represented the good aspects of the primary object. That Hendrix was symbiotically fused with the guitar is an understatement. He even began to sleep with his instrument. To play the guitar was the one and only thing Hendrix desired. Only by playing the guitar could he control and release the energy of the bad objects he had internalized and repressed. [At times, however, it was apparent that this repressed energy was overwhelming, causing Hendrix to smash his guitar on stage, symbolically destroying the good object.] By using drugs, Hendrix was able to internalize the bad aspects of the primary object and thus preserve its external good aspects.

In simpler terms, Hendrix used the guitar to compensate for the loss of the primary object (mother). The guitar specifically, and his music in general, became a compensatory representation of the good aspects of the primary object. "The women in Jimi's songs are primarily angels and Madonna's. Many appear to be his mother Lucille invoked as a savior and redeemer" (Shapiro & Glebbeek, 1990, p.226). In order to protect these good aspects, or to preserve the guitar as good and pleasurable, Hendrix took drugs. His drug use effected the internalization and repression of the bad objects. In order to relieve the tension from the repression of the bad objects, Hendrix played the guitar in an attempt to control their release.

After he achieved fame, Hendrix' early pathology became increasingly apparent. He would alternate between hyperanimation, as if he were possessed of some superhuman energy, and lethargy and withdrawal. More than likely his drug use enhanced this cycle. Nevertheless, towards the end of his life, Hendrix seemed increasingly more exhausted and withdrawn, as well as confused. For the first time in his life, he lacked energy on stage. His last recording from a concert at the Isle of Wight displays a despair and urgency that would be readily apparent to anyone who has worked with the deeply pathological. It is almost a cry for release from psychic bondage to his internalized bad objects.

Perhaps unconsciously, he did commit suicide—a last ditch attempt to destroy the bad objects trapped inside himself.

The Case of Elvis Presley

Elvis Aaron Presley was born to a poor white southern family. Elvis was the younger of a set of twins. His brother who preceded him by a few minutes was stillborn. Elvis' young parents were devastated by the loss of their first child and had not realized that there were two babies. Consequently, Elvis' normal birth was greeted with much happiness.

By most accounts Elvis was well cared for and perhaps even spoiled. Although his family was poor, Elvis' parents, especially his mother, indulged him. Elvis grew up as a polite and respectful child. Because of the Presley's poverty, the family lived in close proximity and Elvis shared a bed with his parents until his teens. Elvis remained close to his parents throughout his life. According to Hammontree (1985),

> An often repeated part of the Elvis legend is his closeness to his parents. It is quite true that a strong bond existed among them. Vernon Presley stated after Elvis' death "It is hard to describe the feelings Elvis, his mother, and I had for each other. The three of us formed our own private world"...This closeness was a powerful influence in Elvis' life. (p. 7)

Elvis was also close to his extended family and surrounded himself with family and friends throughout his life. In fact, Elvis generally preferred to stay at home surrounded by a retinue of family and friends rather than going into the world outside. This pattern of having 'gatherings' at his home began when Elvis was a young man and continued until his death.

Elvis did not stand out as a teenager or a young man with the exception of his clothes and hair. Later on Elvis' clothes, hairstyle and use of makeup would lend him some flair and distinction. Rather than seeking popularity or isolation at school, Elvis had his own group of friends with whom he spent time. He had picked up the guitar a few years earlier and enjoyed playing and singing for his family and friends. Much of Elvis' interest in music can be traced to his family's involvement with a somewhat charismatic church sect in which strong emotions would be experienced and expressed during the service. Music was an integral part of the church service. It is, therefore, not surprising to find that for Elvis, the expression of emotion was intimately related to music. Elvis eventually got a chance to make a record. Due in part to talent, luck, and the marketability of a white singer who could successfully imitate black music, Elvis began a meteoric rise to stardom.

Off-stage Elvis was shy and withdrawn. Once on stage, however, Elvis became possessed by the emotion of the music resulting in the gyrations that were to become his trademark. An interesting aspect of Elvis' musical career was his association with his manager Tom Parker. While Elvis was generally soft-spoken, generous, hard-working and respectful of those around him, Parker was "an obese, crude, cigar-smoking man" (Hammontree, 1985, p.15). It was reported that Parker hated music and musicians and was clearly in it only for the money. Elvis, on the other hand, was fairly indifferent to money matters and somewhat of a musical perfectionist, concerned primarily with putting on a good show for his fans.

Elvis connected with audiences in such a way as to guarantee that their interaction became almost a mystical experience of oneness. No doubt Elvis' ability to communicate and bond with his fans accounts for his tremendous popularity. It is said that Elvis lived to perform and that audience contact recharged and invigorated him. It is strange, therefore, that for close to ten years, Elvis gave up live performances to make movies. From 1960 to 1970 Elvis made over 30 movies at an astonishing rate of 2-3 per year. At the end of this period Elvis returned to live performances, both in Las Vegas and on tour around the country (Cotten, 1985).

During the 1970's Elvis maintained his touring schedule. When he was not performing, he lived at Graceland with a large extended family made up of relations and a retinue of close friends. As Hammontree (1985) comments,

> Elvis' intense need to surround himself with the familiar
> ironically contributed a destructive element to his life: he
> was too much insulated from reality...leading a kind of
> fantasy existence without financial or household worries
> of any kind. (p. 28)

It is sometime during Elvis' "fantasy existence" that he
began to use drugs. Although no exact date for the beginning of Elvis' drug use has been recorded it is possible to
guess that his drug use probably became increasingly frequent throughout his career. Elvis had a paradoxical attitude
towards drugs. He was strongly opposed to the use of illegal
drugs. Yet, at the same time, he compulsively used a wide
variety of prescription drugs which included amphetamines,
tranquilizers, and steroids. Hammontree (1985) describes
this split in Elvis' view of drugs,

> An irony was Elvis' intense opposition to recreational
> drugs, often called 'street' drugs...He thought the use of
> recreational drugs despicable. When his stepbrother Rick
> Stanley became a heroin addict, Elvis expressed anger
> and frustration at Stanley's use of the drug. Stanley con-
> sidered it astonishing that Elvis would take him to task,
> force him to enter a drug rehabilitation center to detox-
> ify, while Elvis was at the same time daily taking large
> doses of tranquilizers, pain-killing drugs, and stimu-
> lants...Elvis rationalized his chemical dependence as ac-
> ceptable because his drugs were all prescription drugs.
> In his view, taking prescription drugs bore no relation-
> ship to drug addiction. (p. 90)

Elvis became very knowledgeable about the drugs he
took and probably had a good intellectual understanding of
the long-term side-effects of his drug use. Nevertheless, this
intellectual knowledge did nothing to reduce Elvis' drug
consumption, although it no doubt served to give Elvis the
illusion of control of his habit.

Beginning in the 1970's, Elvis' health began to deterio-
rate. In addition to his physical weakening, Elvis also began
to have less energy and to become emotionally detached.
Although he was hospitalized a number of times, Elvis insisted on maintaining his exhausting touring schedule. It can
be speculated that the worse Elvis felt, the more drugs he
took to maintain his ability to perform. Finally, on the morn-

ing of August 16, 1977, Elvis' body and perhaps his mind, could no longer stand the strain.

Elvis demonstrated many characteristics common to compulsive drug users. At first, it appears that Elvis' relatively stable family life and good relationship with his mother and father would contraindicate the development of a drug habit. Closer scrutiny, however, reveals that Elvis may have suffered early object trauma. A little known fact is that Elvis' father was arrested and jailed on a check forgery charge when Elvis was three years old (Cotten, 1985). Elvis' father was in prison for three years during a crucial period in Elvis' development. Given the fact that Elvis was already regarded as special by his mother and pampered almost beyond the means of his family's modest income, the loss of his father during his infancy resulted in a strong identification with his mother. Elvis' obvious latent homosexuality, evident from his use of makeup, clothes and intimacy with his closest male friends (whom Elvis kept around him at all times) are signs of his mother-identification. Elvis remained fixated at the separation-individuation stage of development. While Elvis was driven to succeed and try new adventures, he worked diligently to maintain a constant emotional environment in which he was nurtured and cared for in every way. Like a small child who wanders away from its mother for a moment, only to run back and make sure she is still there, Elvis would strike out on tour, make movies, travel to Hawaii and then turn back to his familiar environment for support. Elvis brought this familiar environment with him at all times. At first it consisted of his parents. Later, after the death of his mother, Elvis surrounded himself with a retinue of male friends, family members and hanger-ons whose job it was to keep Elvis' emotional life stable and unchanging. Whether he was in Memphis, Hawaii, or Hollywood, Elvis was always in a situation which was controlled and stable.

The loss of his mother was an extreme blow to Elvis and it can be guessed that his drug use escalated after her death. Drugs came to play a role in the maintenance of a constant environment around Elvis in a more reliable way than his family and friends. The main advantage was that drugs (possibly along with musical performing) maintained Elvis' internal psychic environment, allowing Elvis to be in control of his affective states.

Elvis displayed primitive defenses such as splitting. His views on illegal and prescription drugs is a clear case as was his relationship with his manager Tom Parker. Elvis was also capable of demonstrating narcissistic rage, although he could not be deemed a true narcissist (Dodes, 1990). Elvis could very easily put himself into the position of the 'common man' and sought his approval. This attitude came out in his great effort to put on a good performance, even when it drove him to physical collapse. Elvis' concerts, and indeed much of his interaction with others often included the distribution of gifts. This gift distribution was reminiscent of Elvis' childhood which was marked by much gift-giving by his mother (Cotten, 1985).

Elvis' mother-identification may have also been responsible for his popularity and the almost mystical experience of his concert presence. As a great all-powerful mother figure, Elvis could induce his fans to a religious-regressed state of infancy marked by hysterical ecstasy and a sense of identification with someone greater than oneself. This is the same feeling an infant has towards its mother which Elvis was able to recreate over and over again for his fans. Elvis' sexuality also seems to have had a peculiar tinge of motherliness to it, being more related to inclusion in his extended family than phallic-narcissist penetration as seen in so many other rock stars.

Elvis' life is truly fertile ground for the psychopathographer. Although many other aspects of Elvis' life would make for an interesting psychoanalytic exploration, this will be left for another essay. It is enough to comment that Elvis' compulsive drug use had its beginnings in his arrested object relations development and that Elvis' object relations dynamics are similar to those of other compulsive drug users.

Anaclitic Amphetamine-Using Women

This case example comes from an interesting paper by Lidz, Lidz and Rubenstein (1976). In this paper, the authors describe an anaclitic syndrome related to drug use and other compensatory symptoms. Five case histories of female adolescent drug users are presented. These cases are fascinating both in the level of detail on the family histories of the young women and the striking similarities in the phenomenology of each case.

In order to outline and support the points of the present text, the cases will divided into two groups. The first group, consisting of three of the cases presented in the paper, will describe a basic, composite syndrome related to amphetamine use. Two other cases in the same study will demonstrate more unusual, extreme features of the syndrome. A brief summary of the family histories and the object relations constellations will be presented here. For a full reading of the cases the reader is directed to the original paper.

The cases of Oona L., Nancy C., and Helen L. will be presented as a composite. Indeed, the histories, symptoms and phenomenology of these cases are very similar, differing in only a few small details. Each of these patients were in early-to-middle adolescence when their histories were taken. All three young women were confirmed amphetamine abusers and had taken many other substances as well. Amphetamines, however, were the drug of choice for these patients who reported that the drug relieved feelings of depression and emptiness. These three patients also presented what was characterized as borderline or slightly psychotic symptoms and were suicidal to varying degrees. A description of Oona L. will serve to give a flavor of the diagnosis of each of these three patients.

Oona, a 16 year old girl, had used a number of different drugs in large amounts, but had increasingly begun to rely on methedrine as her drug of choice. In addition to her use of drugs, Oona also had personality problems such as a tendency toward paranoia and fantasy life. Nevertheless, Oona was able to communicate well with others, capable of form-

ing friendships, and seemed fairly intelligent. Oona was ad-
mitted to the hospital as an in-patient because of her increasing paranoid fears and suicidal tendencies. Lidz, Lidz, and
Rubenstein's (1976) description of Oona could possibly be
applied to all the girls in the study. She was characterized as
'waif-like', drawing other people to her through this de-
meanor. Both the clinical impression and psychological
testing indicated fright, despair and suicidal tendencies. The
psychological testing also gave an impression of
schizophrenia, but this diagnosis was not confirmed.

The girls' parents were without exception disorganized.
Their fathers were generally unavailable or somehow removed from the families. The fathers were also occasional
drug users, sexually promiscuous, and in some cases seductive towards their daughters. All the fathers presented elements of a narcissistic personality disorder. Nancy C.'s father is illustrative of the typical father of these patients. He
appeared rather intimate and seductive towards Nancy, who
reported that she had slept and took showers with him until
the age of seven. At the time of her hospitalization Nancy's
father would touch and kiss her quite a bit during his visits.
Nancy had some degree of awareness of her father's pathology (as did her brother who was a heroin addict).

The mothers were also not generally available to their
children on an affective level and likely to be depressed and
needy. Oona L.'s mother was typical. She attempted to play
the role of a loving mother, but was incapable of giving anything to her children. She was unable to set limits, often used
the children as confidants, and was generally needy towards
them. Oona's mother was also a 'heavy' user of tranquilizers.
She had become depressed during her pregnancy with Oona
and had remained in a depressed state for at least a year after Oona was born.

The mothers all had difficulty showing love or affection
to their daughters, and setting limits for them. They often
appeared unconcerned about their daughters' behavior with
regard to drugs and sex. The mothers were often disorganized, hostile, promiscuous and used drugs themselves. All
of the mothers had infantile characters and treated their
daughters like a parent. The daughters were expected to take

care of the mothers, who took on dependent roles in relationship to their children.

When the patients entered puberty, or during latency, the fathers became even more emotionally removed, either due to remarriage, withdrawal of affectionate behavior, or through a general withdrawal from the family. During this time period the mothers became increasingly dependent upon the daughters. As soon as the patients entered into adolescence they became involved in sexualized relationships with males on whom they became intensely dependent. This excessive dependency generally caused the males to end the relationships. The end of these relationships marked the beginning of a period of serious drug use and sexual promiscuity. Due to heavy amphetamine use, the patients eventually decompensated to the point of acute psychiatric illness or attempted suicide, at which time they were hospitalized. Helen L.'s case is representative of this pattern.

Helen first began to use amphetamines at 14 because she thought she was overweight. Interestingly enough, her father had a hatred for fat people. It is likely that Helen's envy of thin, sleek girls was related to her father's attitudes. Helen developed an intensely dependent relationship with a boy a few years older than her. Not only did she gratify him sexually, but she sought to spend all her time with him as well. She demanded his attention, was possessive and overly jealous. This was apparently too much for the boy and he broke off the relationship. The boyfriend worked as a bartender and

> ...was heavily into drugs. In order to go along with his crowd, Helen started snorting methedrine. She was soon hospitalized with a methedrine psychosis...At times, she was flagrantly promiscuous. Ever since her suicidal attempt she had a fear of sleeping alone, related to a dread of death. She continued to have frequent suicidal urges, and believed that ultimately she would kill herself. (pp. 333-334)

The composite picture created from these cases shows a pathology of object relations development. It is extremely clear that object relations development in these three patients did not proceed normally and that this can be traced to an insufficient relationship of the infants with their parents. All the mothers were unavailable to their infants. The patients were unable to integrate or internalize the good aspects of their primary objects. The mothers were unable to modulate the transitional object phase of development for their daughters. As a result each patient suffered from anaclitic depression. Because these patients did not successfully resolve the transitional object phase, they remained somewhat in symbiosis with their mothers. Later in life, there was clear evidence of rather nebulous self-object boundaries. The fathers were not able to play their roles in facilitating the child's individuation from the mother. This later was evident in the weak triangulation (or oedipalization) of the parent-child relationships. During the original oedipal stage of development, the fathers compensated for the lack of mothering. The patients, who were not strongly individuated from their mothers, became strongly attached to their fathers. The fathers did not play a normal oedipal role but instead were expected to fulfill anaclitic needs. Later, in adolescence, when oedipal conflicts were reactivated, the fathers were unavailable. Therefore, the patients sought out compensatory objects in the form of a boyfriend. The relationships with these boyfriends were only superficially oedipal in that the relationships were sexual and with males who were sometimes older than the patients. The compensatory nature of the relationships was soon revealed in the extreme dependency of the patients upon their boyfriends. The boyfriends almost certainly compensated for the father, who in turn compensated for the mother. Another way of conceptualizing the dynamics of these patients is to say that the oedipal conflict with the father was mixed up with the preoedipal anaclitic needs of the patients for mothering. These patients reported that having sex was less interesting to them than having someone who would hold them and be with them at night. For instance,

> Nancy, then began to sleep with men simply to be held and because of her fear of sleeping alone. She did not care who the man was, or whether she knew him or not. (p. 328)

Clearly the boyfriends were used to provide nurturing and mothering. When the boyfriends ended the relationships, the patients sought out more reliable compensation and began to use drugs. Although some of the patients became sexually promiscuous at this time, this was a secondary compensation which probably served to keep the patients in a community of drug users. The drugs now became the true compensatory device. Drugs turned out to be superior to either boyfriend or father as compensatory objects. Unlike a boyfriend who cannot tolerate dependence, drugs foster this state in their users. Drugs also more closely represent the longed for maternal care in both its gratifying and frustrating aspects.

Although all five cases presented by Lidz, Lidz and Rubenstein share similar pathological phenomenology, two of the cases contain additional material which is of interest. These cases are those of Sarah A. and Gail T. While the family histories of these two patients are similar to the other three cases discussed above, they are different in that their fathers actually died. The death of the father led to a more profound pathology. This is evident from a brief description as in the case of Sarah A.

> Sarah A. entered the hospital at the age of 18 after having spent eight months in the counterculture, living in numerous pads, heavily involved with drugs, particularly intravenous methedrine, and sleeping with virtually any man who wanted her. She was the only member of the series [of cases] who was clearly a "speed freak". (pp. 329-330)

For Sarah A. the almost complete lack of a father caused her to seek greater compensation and then lapse into greater decompensation. This is apparent when Sarah A.'s first sexual relationship is examined,

> ...at 16 she became infatuated and sexually involved with a music teacher who was older than her parents, an intense experience that lasted for six months. When he dropped her, she felt abandoned but soon took up with a musician in his 30s, and started using "speed" with him. (p. 331)

Sarah A. had a relationship with a man who was old enough to be her father, while Gail T. had a relationship with an older male soon after her father's death. Both of these patients had sought gratification of their anaclitic needs from their fathers because the mothers had not been available. Therefore, the actual loss of the father was experienced as a preoedipal object loss. In these two cases the decompensation to a grave pathological condition seems to have occurred more quickly and with greater severity than in the other three cases. For instance, Gail T. subsequently attempted suicide on the anniversary of her father's death, which led to her hospitalization. Gail also used LSD along with amphetamines, which may have been related to a belated mourning process. Sarah A. appeared to show the most overt borderline characteristics of the group. She lived more 'on the edge' and seemed to require more stimulus in order to experience affect,

> She told of her life in a succession of pads, often with confirmed addicts, criminals, and drug dealers. She narrowly escaped death on several occasions, as when she stepped in front of a man just as another man, who she knew had previously committed murder, was about to shoot him. She found the exciting, dangerous existence pleasurable as it made her feel alive. (p. 331)

Although Sarah A. took up with confirmed criminals, put herself into extremely dangerous situations, and was generally impulsive, she also had another side to her personality,

> She was welcomed in various pads and communes because she was fun to be with when stimulated by drugs, and she was a good cook who was also willing to care for other people's children. (p. 331)

This suggests some level of splitting, which is not surprising given Sarah A.'s borderline characteristics.

The Successful Analysis of a Heroin Addict

Berthelsdorf (1976) describes in detail his analysis of a nineteen-year-old male college student who was addicted to heroin. The patient was seen for four years of analytic work, which ranged from 3 to 7 days per week. This case is interesting in that it was successful and is almost an ideal model of the use of classical psychoanalysis in the treatment of drug addiction.

The patient, Don, was referred to Berthelsdorf because of his addiction. An initial *House-Tree-Person* test revealed object relations deficits with regard to the mother. Don's family history was somewhat scant. His family consisted of a father, mother and an elder sister. The family appeared to be intact and not disorganized. There was some indication, however, that Don's mother may have had drug use problems herself, and that she may have been emotionally distant.

Don's drug use started when his mother gave him a tranquilizer and showed him where they were kept. He immediately began using these drugs without telling anyone about it. Don soon began to sell drugs and built up a secret bank account from these endeavors. He eventually was arrested for selling drugs and was expelled from school. Nevertheless, Don studied at home and was able to earn a high school diploma and gain entrance into college. Don did quite well in college despite his drug use and was highly intelligent.

Don was at times markedly self-critical and would have outbursts of hostility towards others. Nevertheless, he did not appear disaffected and could express both sadness and rage during his treatment. His affect, however, was somewhat labile. Don's psychopathology clearly demonstrated both preoedipal object relations and oedipal lines of development. In an initial session he described a dream that gives an indication of both lines of conflict:

> In the first part he was with his father, who had his arm about Don, giving a sense of comfort and intimacy. In the second part, Don was buying some heroin from an untrustworthy drug pusher, and felt he was putting himself in the hands of a man who could betray him. That man indeed had recently sold Don some very poor-quality marijuana. (Berthelsdorf, 1976, p. 170)

This dream shows an oedipal conflict with an underlying anaclitic component. Berthelsdorf responded to the dream by commenting that Don needed a comforting, nurturing relationship with other people including his analyst, but that he feared the consequences of such a relationship. This interpretation was confirmed later when Don brought up a fantasy of performing oral sex on his analyst. Berthelsdorf's interpretation focused on the underlying meaning rather than the overt content of the fantasy. This deeper meaning was that the analyst was a nursing mother and that Don was a suckling infant, wanting the pleasurable feeling from the analyst that he had been receiving from the heroin. This interpretation proved to pivotal in deepening the analysis.

Don's anaclitic needs for nurturing were also accompanied by separation-individuation issues as well as problems in maintaining a sense of object constancy. Don also showed some signs of defensive splitting. For instance, he had a strong need to be with other people, but subsequently felt trapped by his relationships with them. Also, when Don was parting with an acquaintance, he would compulsively want to know when he would see the person again, even if it was someone he did not like. Don also felt very strongly that his life with his drug-using friends was at odds with his life with his parents. It was as if "...he had to cope with two alien worlds, each to be denied the existence in the other" (p. 171).

Overall, Don's addiction can be understood as a result of his identification with his mother. This identification was originally carried out by Don taking his mother's drugs. Later, the drugs came to represent, or compensate for his mother. Clearly, Don's addictive pathology was due to a preoedipal problem. Fortunately, Don demonstrated a lack of impulsivity which gave him a reasonably good prognosis with classical psychoanalytic treatment.

Berthelsdorf's strategy in this case can be likened to a replacement of the drug by the analyst. In this strategy the analyst becomes a transitional object for the addicted patient. Compensating affects and the control of affect are slowly transferred to the analyst, and then even more slowly internalized by the patient. In Don's case, he became pacified after the initial hour, assuming all of his problems were solved, as if by magic. He also understood the analyst, however, as dangerous, threatening to upset the status quo. Don, therefore, sought out more comfort or pacification from Berthelsdorf during the analytic hour, while continuing to use drugs between therapy sessions.

Eventually, the process of analysis became extremely intense as the analyst took on more of the object role than the drug. Berthelsdorf began at this time to see Don seven days a week. The object relations characteristics of the analysis became more obvious, as Don regressed in therapy to a ravenous infant, feeding off the analyst. In this state Don was able to express anger at Berthelsdorf, while maintaining a feeling of security from his destructive urge to swallow the analyst.

It is interesting to note the oedipal conflict in Don's case. The oedipal situation provided a barometer of Don's development throughout his analysis. Don's relationships moved during his analysis from decidedly dyadic modes to more triangular ones. In the beginning of the analytic work, Don's oedipal conflict was presented more in terms of anaclitic needs, which were similar to those seen in the five cases of female amphetamine addicts described previously. As Don progressed, his conflicts became increasingly triangulated. For example, early in his analysis Don recalled his first sexual experience,

> Don had his first heterosexual experience as a freshman in college, after years of attempts and failures caused by the loss of erection. On this occasion he was staying overnight with a fellow and his girlfriend. He decided to go to the bathroom just as the two were finishing the act of intercourse and he was passing by their bed. He stopped, humbly asked the young man if "it" would be all right with him and the girl. They agreed and Don succeeded. Subsequently he was only occasionally concerned about his impotence. (p. 179)

This experience clearly shows Don's inability to resolve separation-individuation issues. Similar sexual experiences have also been reported by other compulsive drug using patients (Fine, 1972; Savitt, 1954). Don could not achieve potency under normal conditions, indicating a weak identification with the father. Don is unable to be a rival and win the woman/mother for himself, in essence to be on his own. Instead, he approaches a weak father-figure and "humbly" requests that his desires be gratified. There is no need to separate from the mother because the father-figure at this point is like the mother, magically taking care of the infant's needs. It is not surprising that Don was preoccupied about homosexuality, as his identification with a male father-figure was a thin screen for his symbiotic relationship to the mother. Compare the above scenario to a similar scene which occurred later in Don's analysis. He was visiting some friends, a couple and gave them some heroin. The women injected herself and went out of the room to have sex with her boyfriend. After they had left, Don gave himself an injection,

> ....I learned that he was at that moment reminded of his mother and father leaving for an evening, and of their giving him his "reward for bravery!"...The next thing he knew, his friend was giving him mouth-to-mouth respiration, and someone else was shaking and slapping him, talking to him to keep him awake. He was told he had stopped breathing...Over a year later a final fragment of this episode came to light; the girl had exposed her breasts to him when she gave herself the injection just before leaving the room; and he could hear them making love in the next room as he gave himself all the heroin he had left. (p. 181)

This description confirms the symbolism of the couple as representing father and mother. This time, however, Don was more on his own, more individuated. The father-figure this time did not magically fulfill Don's needs, but instead took the mother for himself. Don was in a more classical oedipal position in this situation. Although, the mother-figure was clearly present and available (with breasts exposed), Don could not possess her without conflict. The father-figure was now a potent rival unlike the previous scenario. This possibly engendered feelings of rage and guilt in Don. His response to these feelings was to take an overdose of heroin. This use of drugs was, therefore, both an attempt to possess the mother (through the incorporation of her substitute, heroin) and an attempt to control intolerable affect (guilt and rage).

Still later in the analysis the oedipal conflict became central to the treatment as the analyst was seen more as the father in the transference. Berthelsdorf reports that this stage occurred after 360 hours of therapy. This stage of the analysis was characterized by the analyst being experienced more as a competitor or rival.

Eventually, Don was able to resolve his separation-individuation conflict, resulting in the ability to relinquish the use of drugs. It seems that Don was then able to work with his oedipal conflict to some degree and achieve a healthy integration of appropriate parental objects into his personality.

Summary and Conclusions

These case histories of compulsive drug users point quite clearly to a pathology of object relations. Most of the compulsive drug users described in this chapter demonstrate defenses like splitting, omnipotent narcissism and other borderline-level defenses. Compulsive drug users can seem to lack object constancy and be highly self-critical. In most cases, the drug itself is used as a reactivated transitional object in an attempt to repair early object relations deficits. From the cases cited above, it seems as if these early object relations deficits can be traced to somewhat specific dynamics between the infant and its parents.

The mothers of compulsive drug users generally appear weak and depressed and have many unmet needs of their own. Their children are starved emotionally and the transitional object phase is not successfully negotiated. Yet, these mothers cling to their children with the hope that their offspring will somehow magically take care them and alleviate their pain. This effectively prevents the separation of the child from its mother. In Winnicott's terminology, these are not 'good enough mothers'.

Nevertheless, the blame does not entirely rest with the mother. In many instances the mother's problems are caused or exacerbated by the fathers. These men are often physically or emotionally unavailable. When they are present, they are often narcissistic, expecting both mother and child to gratify their needs. The fathers, therefore, do not fulfill their role in helping their children separate from the mother. In some cases, the father takes over the mothering role for the child, but usually is emotionally distant or uses the role to get the child to gratify his narcissistic needs. As a result, the apparent oedipal conflicts seen among compulsive drug users often thinly veil earlier object relations conflicts. In other words, the child tries to resolve its object relations needs (caused by inadequate mothering) through a relationship with the father. When this fails, the child (or possibly by now young adult) may turn to other people or fetish-like objects to mediate their internal object relations conflicts.

Clearly, environmental influences come into play during this time. If the child is in an environment where the use of drugs is accepted or tolerated, they will be more likely to use drugs to compensate for their problems. From the review of the literature in Chapter Two, we know that most drug prevention efforts attempt to intervene at this point. Unfortunately, the personality problems underlying the compulsive use of drugs are already well-established. Even if the child were dissuaded from using drugs through educational or other preventive methods, it is highly likely they would turn to some other destructive and compulsive behavior using fetish-like objects.

If the fetish-like object is a drug, a powerful, temporary defensive repair of the object relations deficits is effected following the cycle I outlined in Chapter Four. This drug use becomes compulsive as the physiological properties of the drug catalyzes the borderline-level defenses. This leaves the compulsive drug user to live out a disaffected, dysphoric and pathologically repetitive existence dominated by the good and bad aspects of the drug.

Chapter Six

Compulsive Drug Use—Conclusions

An object relations understanding of drug use leads to two conclusions. The first conclusion is that occasional use by 'normal' individuals is probably not psychologically damaging and not likely to lead to permanent psychological pathology. The catch, of course, is the determination of normalcy. In a strict sense everyone carries the seeds of pathology. Nevertheless, recent research has shown that those who try drugs usually do not suffer any ill effects and may even benefit from the experience (Shedler & Block, 1990). Most persons with satisfactory object relations will probably not feel the need to compulsively use drugs, much as normal adults no longer need transitional objects from their childhood. This is true even for drugs that are highly addictive. An often quoted example is that most of the soldiers who became addicted to heroin in Vietnam gave up the habit once they returned to America (Zinberg, 1975). Once they were away from the stress of the war the need to use drugs diminished. For an individual who has a strong ego formation and mature object relations, experimental drug use may have positive benefits, including increased self-awareness of early object states (Grof, 1985). Like Freud, this individual is not likely to become a habitual user of hard drugs (Jones, 1961, p. 55).

On the other hand, the compulsive drug user is more likely to have had a history of poor object relations. An individual with poor object relations, a weak ego formation,

narcissistic disturbances and a history of introjective depression is likely to begin to use drugs as reactivated transitional objects. Instead of developing good object relations,
this individual may instead use drugs. At first his outer relationships may even improve as he is accepted into a group of
drug using peers (Bentler, 1987). But this is likely to be a
transitory phenomena. Eventually, if the individual's use of
drugs increases, ego destruction, schizoid pathology and
even suicide may be consequences.

Of course, these two scenarios of the normal and pathological are extremes. Most people probably fall somewhere
in between and it is important for the therapist to delineate
the drug *abuser* from the experimental user (Gottesfeld,
Caroff & Lieberman, 1973). As of yet there is no reliable way
to determine who is hiding early object relations pathology
on a mass scale. Therefore, drug use remains a game of psychological 'Russian Roulette'. Like Pandora's box, drug use
presents a situation where the ills inside are not known until
the box is opened and it is too late. On the other hand,
opening the Pandora's box of drugs in a controlled and supportive setting, could give individuals a chance to find and
work through hidden pathology. For instance, Ling and
Buckman's (1965) description of the successful treatment of
frigidity with a combination of LSD and Ritalin (see below)
is a good example of a positive use for drugs. Although the
idea of this type of treatment is now a bit wild for most
practitioners in the US (and also illegal), it has been, or is
being, tried with reported success elsewhere (Andrizsky,
1989; Grof, 1985; Villoldo, 1977).

Treatment

The early history of the psychoanalytic treatment of compulsive drug use is valuable for both its historical perspective
and its relevance to modern modes of therapy. Many early
analysts believed that compulsive drug use, like the psychoses, was not amenable to analysis. The early psychoanalysts who wrote on the treatment of compulsive drug users
unanimously reported that these patients are difficult to

treat. Most recommended treatment in an inpatient setting. This would allow for the medical treatment of the effects of the drug, leading to abstinence. A patient under the influence of a drug was not felt to be a prime analytic candidate until he stopped using the drug or began to use it in a controlled fashion. It was thought that the inpatient setting should not be too controlling, rigid, or punitive, however, as the patient may experience this as a punishment which might exacerbate his condition. Some psychoanalysts, like H. Rosenfeld (1965), felt that the psychoanalytic method could work with compulsive drug users. Other, like Knight (1938), believed the analytic approach to treatment, in these cases, must be modified.

For more modern psychoanalytic clinicians, the main initial task of therapy with drug users is for the therapist to maintain a supportive neutral presence while helping the drug user to re-establish healthy object relations dynamics. It is important for the therapist to maintain this presence throughout the chaos engendered by transference and countertransference phenomena. Charles-Nicolas, Valleur and Tonnelier (1982) express this eloquently,

> A partir de la trame imaginaire et symbolique que nous tissons pour tenter d'organiser le chaos, nous nous heurtons á la course du toxicomane aprés l'inatteignable réel qui n'est pas sans rappeler la quéte de l'object primordial. (p. 209)
> [In our effort to organize chaos in our imaginary and symbolic frame, we hurl ourselves along the course of addiction towards the unobtainable reality that recalls the existence of the primordial object.]

For compulsive drug users, it would be expected that treatment efforts which engender a transference relationship with a positive role model would be the most successful. If the course of treatment proceeds well, the therapist will take on the transitional object aspects of the drug. As suggested by Brill (1977), a relationship with a therapist who represents a consistent good transitional object may have the best chance at compensating for the use of drugs. Only when this relationship is established is there a chance to release or in-

tegrate the bad internalized object representations. As
Fairbairn says,

> At the same time there is now little doubt in my mind
> that the release of the bad object from the unconscious is
> one of the chief aims which the psychotherapist should
> set himself out to achieve...The bad object can only be
> released, however, if the analyst has become established
> as a sufficiently good·object. (1952, p. 70)

The therapist in the role of a transitional object can help
an individual attain a controlled release of the bad internal
object representations. In more modern parlance, this would
be seen as healing the split between the good and bad object
representations. It would, therefore, not be surprising to find
that treatment efforts incorporating some level of transference or identification with the therapist would have a high
degree of short-term success. As Dodes (1990) says,

> ...the use of Alcoholics Anonymous and its central con-
> cept of a "higher power" may be understood as exam-
> ples of a search for an idealized object and an omnipo-
> tent transitional object, whose powers are utilized in ex-
> change for a loss of power entailed in giving up the
> drug. Likewise, the therapist or analyst may also be
> quickly created or perceived to be such an idealized nar-
> cissistic object, leading to the rapid achievement of drug
> abstinence. (p. 417)

Programs such as the twelve-step or co-dependency
groups which include elements designed to bond drug
abusers to a positive environment and role models may
work for this reason. Experienced therapists like Khantzian
(1990) and Wurmser (1985) have suggested that psychodynamic treatment be supplemented by involvement in self-
help groups. Although it is recognized that some severely
pathological patients may not tolerate the self-help approach, many patients will derive benefit from this type of
supportive, contained environment. Also, as Khantzian
(1990) reports, self-help groups like AA (Alcoholics
Anonymous), NA (Narcotics Anonymous) or CA (Cocaine
Anonymous) force compulsive drug users to face the defensive denial and narcissism associated with their drug problem. Both the admission of addiction and the storytelling of

drug experiences by patients in self-help groups may play a valuable psychodynamic role in overcoming these defenses. Nevertheless, without the deep insight engendered in psychoanalytic therapy, the success of the self-help approach alone may be transitory. Without the support of an external agency (e.g. a supportive therapist or self-help group) the drug user will likely fall back into his old habits. Because the addict has relied on an external, reactivated transitional object for support, he does not necessarily have the motivation to internalize this support. This internalization comes about through introspective psychoanalytic work, which requires some ability to tolerate painful affect (Federn, 1952). Of course, this is why psychotherapeutic treatment with compulsive drug users is reported to be extremely difficult (Fine, 1972; Wurmser, 1974). For this reason, it is perhaps best to do introspective work in combination with psychotherapies or self-help modalities which provide some external support. Although there is no good evidence which delineates the effectiveness of different types of drug treatment programs, this type of multimodal approach may have the best chance of success (Schiffer, 1988). Wurmser (1985, 1987) suggests a comprehensive approach to treatment along these lines, which he calls a "combination treatment" (1985, p. 95). Wurmser conceptualizes this approach as follows,

> Psychoanalysis has a great deal to offer in a situation of despair. But again as in the early days of Freud's work we often have to combine the analytic, uncovering approach with other measures. It is as if the *vertical* approach of analysis needed to be supplemented by a *horizontal* approach. (Wurmser, 1985, p. 164)

Wurmser goes on to describe a patient who in addition to analysis five days a week, was also concurrently treated with counter-phobic behavioral methods, AA meetings, Antabuse, and, for a short time, antidespressant drugs. Wurmser does not believe that every type of approach is needed in all cases. Nevertheless, in his view, the successful treatment of compulsive drug users through analysis alone is the exception, not the rule. The analytic part of the treatment may also need to be slightly modified, with the analyst providing some suggestions. The classical analytic stance of the analyst, however, should not change. This does not mean that the analyst's technical neutrality should equate to being cool, aloof, or indifferent. Instead, the analyst should maintain his neutral stance while simultaneously maintaining a "strong emotional presence" (Wurmser, 1985, p. 94). Khantzian (1990), while agreeing with much of Wurmser's position, suggests that the therapeutic stance should be much more supportive, providing structure and containment.

Other psychoanalysts have reported successful treatment outcomes through the sole use of psychoanalysis (Berthelsdorf, 1976; Fine, 1972). Berthelsdorf (1976), for instance, does not greatly modify the classical psychoanalytic approach. He does, however, take care not to frustrate the compulsive drug using patient and hence, takes on a more supportive role than is usually found in classical analytic treatment. No doubt level of functioning and motivation play a large role in determining whether or not analysis alone is indicated for a specific patient. Therefore, some generalizations can be made about the treatment of drug users from a more or less psychoanalytic point of view.

For those drug users who are more regressed and present a more overt psychotic or borderline pathology, a regimented, protected environment with a high degree of support may be beneficial in the first stages of therapy in which the users begin to abstain from the drug. As Kernberg (1975) suggests, "...psychotherapeutic treatment may best start out with a period of prolonged hospitalization" (p. 191). This supportive, structured environment can provide assistance and auxiliary functions to the patient's ego as well as suitable (good) external objects. It has also been recommended that sexual issues be addressed in this supportive environment. Healthy sexual strivings should be supported and consensual relations among patients should not be suppressed. After the initial phase of therapy, outpatient treatment may be attempted as long as a high level of support is maintained. (DeAngelis, 1975).

For higher functioning drug users, underlying issues and pathology related to the character of the patient and the drug of choice should be addressed. For instance, introjective depression, rage and lability of affect should be considered in a patient who is addicted to opiates. Likewise, issues of meaninglessness, existential ennui and mourning should be addressed in the user of psychedelics. Stimulant users should be examined with a eye towards underlying depression and feelings of extreme inadequacy. Moreover, in all drug users, defects in object relations should be suspected. Issues related to anaclitic object needs and separation-individuation should be examined. Oedipal conflicts should be carefully scrutinized for underlying preoedipal pathology. The father may have taken over the maternal object role, failed to mediate the separation of the infant from the mother, or both. The therapist should look to his or her own countertransference dynamic with the patient for evidence of defective object relations (Boyer, 1979a, 1983, 1992; Boyer & Giovacchini, 1993; McDougall, 1984, 1985). Additionally, the transference between the patient and the drug of choice should also provide insight into the patient's object relations pathology.

Dodes emphasizes that narcissistic transferences are to be expected in treatment. The therapist may be seen as an omnipotent transitional object, "whose powers are utilized in exchange for the loss of power entailed in giving up the drug" (p. 417). This narcissistic transference can result in a rapid abstinence from drug use because the addict has the power and ego functions of the therapist to help him abstain. Removal of the therapist and his auxiliary ego before the addict has internalized these functions can result in a relapse. As has been mentioned, this quick cure, which Dodes calls a "transference cure", should not be a substitute for a longer course of therapy in which unconscious processes are interpreted in the light of the problem of drug use. The interpretation of drugs as transitional objects may become a central issue in the treatment and understanding of compulsive drug users, giving them insight into their affective states.

Last but certainly not least, the importance of countertransference in treating the compulsive drug user should be emphasized. As the therapist takes over the role of the good external object, he or she may begin to feel treated like a drug. As D. Rosenfeld (1992) reports,

> ...the therapist's most difficult task regarding his countertransference is to stop feeling like, and being, the drug or inanimate object, since this is the role these patients continuously force on him. (p. 209)

When the therapist begins to experience countertransference with the compulsive drug user he or she will begin to feel like an inanimate object, answering the patient mechanically, and speaking according to the patient's wishes. The therapist may then begin to take on an inflexible, rigid attitude and the therapy itself stagnates. D. Rosenfeld (1992) suggests that the therapist can escape the pitfalls of countertransference by engaging in a 'complementary style' of psychotherapy, which consists of taking on a role that is the opposite of what the compulsive drug user experienced from his parents. D. Rosenfeld (1993) also suggests that the countertransference is an important tool for understanding and decoding the early family dynamics of the compulsive drug user. When speaking of the countertransference with his patient George he says,

> ...I understood that these were the types of messages George received daily at home. In other words, I was the object of maddening messages and guilt-generating accusations: the stepmother was doing to me what she did to George every single day. The technical use of the countertransference was very effective in helping me discover the family structure and the sick communication system in which George was ensnared. (1993, p. 224)

From countertransference reactions like these, Rosenfeld was able to formulate more precise interpretations. This use of countertransference phenomenon to guide interpretation has been championed by Boyer (1992).

Prevention

With regard to the prevention of drug use, it is unfortunate that many educational drug abuse prevention efforts use standard informational approaches, or 'scare tactics', which are not effective (Moskowitz, 1983; Pickens, 1985; Wurmser, 1978, 1985, 1987). Some researchers have taken the position that drug abuse prevention should be with children at very young ages (Hawkins, Lishner, Catalano & Howard, 1986; Hawkins, Jenson, Catalano & Lishner, 1988). This especially makes sense from a psychoanalytic viewpoint. What is needed are programs that present the reality about drug use without value laden messages. This should be combined with strong educational and therapeutic practice related to development of positive external object relations.

Psychoanalytic play therapy, Play Analysis (A. Freud, 1946; Klein, 1959) or some form of art therapy (Kramer, 1971; Lowenfeld, 1979; Naumberg, 1973; Ulman & Dachinger, 1975) can be invaluable in correcting and maintaining the object relations health of young children. Luzzatto (1987) has suggested art therapy may be extremely valuable as a treatment modality for compulsive drug users, who might otherwise have a negative therapeutic reaction. While valuable as treatment modalities, these techniques can and should also be used in a prevention context. While not all art therapies are strictly psychoanalytic, they rely without exclusion, on the development of a transference relationship, in which the therapist can be seen as a good and consistent object.

Of course techniques and approaches such as play therapy and psychotherapy cannot take the place of good parenting. The best drug prevention effort would be to provide parenting education to people before they have children. This education effort should include material on the emotional development of children so that potential parents will have a better understanding of the consequences of their actions as parents. While such programs may be expensive in the short term, the amount of money saved in the long term could be tremendous.

General Implications for Society

It is important in a discussion of drug use to take a wider view of the problem. So far, the etiology of the individual drug user has been the focus of the arguments presented here. This focus has followed from the third definition of the psychopathology of drug use given in Chapter Two. It may be useful at this point to touch broadly upon the societal viewpoint implicit in not only this third viewpoint, but the other two as well. Consider the following scenes:

Sometime in the early 1960s a man crossed the border from California into Mexico and went to the town of Tijuana. His purpose was to have a night of drinking and carousing in the border town. Regardless of his intention that night, this man was not a degenerate character. He was a Marine veteran who had seen action in Korea. He had been awarded the purple heart, had an excellent military record and was currently married with two children. Sometime during the evening this veteran was given three or four marijuana cigarettes. Whether he had smoked any marijuana or not is not known. What is known is that when this man arrived at the border drunk, he was thoroughly searched and the marijuana cigarettes were discovered. He was immediately thrown into jail. It was recognized by the court that this man was not a drug dealer and was not a habitual drug user. Nevertheless, sometime later, this man who was a father and a war veteran, was convicted of felony charges of drug possession and sentenced to five years in the penitentiary without the possibility of parole (Smith, 1968).

During roughly the same time period, two psychiatrists who were frustrated with the treatment of frigidity with conventional psychotherapy, embarked on a promising new treatment of the disorder. This treatment involved the administration of LSD-25 and Ritalin (a central nervous system stimulant) together with psychotherapy. In a test case, a women suffering from frigidity without other neurotic or physical complaints was successfully treated in six sessions using the new LSD/psychotherapy technique. In all, sixteen such cases were successfully treated. Although frigidity had been known as notoriously difficult to treat, the psychiatrists felt that "...Given good motivation, superior intelligence, a reasonable stable personality and a cooperative potent spouse, psychotherapy with LSD can help these cases by the recovery of early sexual fantasies or traumatic experiences responsible for symptom formation" (Ling & Buckman, 1965, p. 239).

These two vastly different outcomes of the use of drugs give an idea of the lack of consistency towards drugs and drug use in our society. Although the harshness of marijuana laws in most states have been reduced, LSD psychotherapy is now illegal even under the care of a qualified physician. Therefore, even though there has been some change in our societal view of drug use, we are still confused.

Drug use has historically been a highly emotional issue in America. Even in the very earliest days of the U.S. war on drugs, emotional and hysterical responses often outweighed scientific evidence which did not support the claim that drugs were responsible for a variety of societal ills. For instance, the first clinics for the rehabilitation of opiate addicts which opened in 1919, were closed down a scant four years later. This loss of support for the clinics was largely a result in a change of attitude toward drug users by society. Before 1919, drug addicts were seen as the unfortunate victims of a serious malady. After 1923, the same drug addicts were seen as hardened criminals. Later these attitudes were extended to other drugs. For example, in the middle of the 1930's a government committee heard testimony from Dr. William C. Woodward, legislative counsel for the American Medical Association. Dr. Woodward opposed the passage of a law to make marijuana illegal. The committee's response was to severely question Dr. Woodward's credentials and to criticize him for being uncooperative. Finally he was rebuked for trying to get in the way of something the government wanted to do (Smith, 1968).

Not much has changed since the 1930's. Drug use is still an emotionally charged issue. The only differences are that the government's 'War on Drugs' has taken on an even higher media profile. Nevertheless many scientists have come to agree with Dr. Woodward's lone message. In fact, many in the scientific community advocate the legalization or decriminalization of potent drugs, although this is still a hot topic for debate (Inciardi, 1991; Nadelmann, 1989). There are many reasons why some scientists favor the legalization or decriminalization of drugs. Perhaps the most important reason for those in the psychological community is to once again attempt to understand the problems of compulsive drug users in terms of psychopathology. Without a doubt, a societal view which sees drug users only as criminals impedes this type of understanding.

Although the legalization of drugs is not likely to occur in the near future, Americans collectively continue to consume vast amounts of drugs. The impulse to use drugs is no doubt present to an extreme degree, especially given the statistics on drug use. Yet, this impulse is excluded and severely repressed from societal consciousness. The wish to use drugs is vigorously denied and rigid prescriptions have been established to guide societal authorities. These prescriptions, unfortunately, deny many of the most basic truths regarding drug use by individuals. Many of these so-called authorities suffer from what might be termed reaction-formation symptoms. These can be seen in the health educator who rigidly preaches the evils of drug use, while consuming large amounts of alcohol and coffee, or the appalling number of addicted physicians and nurses. Included in our mass denial of drugs are the reasons driving us to use these substances. For the urban poor, environmental and economic influences undoubtedly play a large role. As this review has indicated, the impact of the family on early intrapsychic development is important among all types of compulsive drug users. The roles of intrapsychic family dynamics have, unfortunately, been all but ignored in much of the sociological and social psychology research on drug use.

Like the Maenads in their wild dance, we are too entranced by our bloody feast to see that it consists of our children. Perhaps on a societal level we will someday be able to take energy away from our defenses against drugs and invest it into insight into the phenomena. Until this happens drug use will continue to be a dangerous, frightening and poorly understood problem.

Bibliography

Abraham, K. (1908). The psychological relations between sexuality and alcoholism. In *Selected Papers on Psycho-Analysis*. London, England: Hogarth Press.

Abraham, K. (1910). Remarks on the psycho-analysis of a case of foot and corset fetishism. In *Selected Papers on Psycho-Analysis*. London, England: Hogarth Press.

Adams-Silvan, A., & Adams, M. (1986). The relation of psychosexual development to the successful exercise of power in a woman ruler: A study of Catherine de Medici. *Psychoanalytic Inquiry, 6*(1), 49-65.

Adler, G. (1986). Psychotherapy of the narcissistic personality disorder patient: Two contrasting approaches. *American Journal of Psychiatry, 143*(4), 430-436.

Almansi, R. J. (1983). On the persistence of very early memory traces in psychoanalysis, myth, and religion. *Journal of the American Psychoanalytical Association, 31*(2), 391-421.

American Psychiatric Association, (1987). *Diagnostic and statistical manual of mental disorders: Third edition - revised.* Washington, DC: American Psychiatric Association.

Andrizsky, W. (1989). Sociopsychotherapeutic functions of Ayahuasca healing in Amazonia. Special Issue:

Shamanism and altered states of consciousness. *Journal of Psychoactive Drugs, 21*(1), 77-89.

Arieti, S. (1967). *The intrapsychic self: Feeling, cognition and creativity in health and mental illness.* New York, NY: Basic Books.

Babst, D. V., Miran, M., & Koval, M. (1976). The relationship between friends' marijuana use, family cohesion, school interest and drug abuse prevention. *Drug Education, 6*(1), 23-40.

Battjes, R. J., & Pickens, R. W. (1988). *Needle sharing among intravenous drug abusers: National and international perspectives. NIDA Research Monograph 80.* U.S. Department of Health and Human Services. (DHHS Publication Number ADM88-1567). Rockville, MD: National Institute of Drug Abuse.

Bentler, P. M. (1987). Drug use and personality in adolescence and young adulthood: Structural models with nonnormal variables. *Child Development, 58,* 65-79.

Beres, D. (1966). Superego and depression. In Lowenstein, R. M., Newman, L. M., Schur, M., & Solnit, A. J. (Eds.). *Psychoanalysis - a general psychology: Essays in honor of Heinz Hartmann.* New York, NY: International Universities Press.

Berman, L. E. A. (1972). The role of amphetamine in the case of hysteria. *Journal of the American Psychoanalytical Association, 20,* 325-340.

Berthelsdorf, S. (1976). Survey of the successful analysis of a young man addicted to heroin. *Psychoanalytic Study of the Child, 31,* 165-191.

Blanck, R., & Blanck, G. (1986). *Beyond ego psychology: Developmental object relations theory.* New York, NY: Columbia University Press.

Blatt, S. J., & Lerner, H. (1983). The psychological assessment of object representation. *Journal of Personality Assessment*, 47(1), 7-28.

Blatt, S.J., Berman, W., Bloom-Feschbach, S., Sugarman, A., Wilber, C., & Kleber, (1984). Psychological assessment of psychopathology in opiate addicts. *Journal of Nervous and Mental Disease*, 172(4), 156-165.

Blatt, S.J., McDonald, C., Sugarman, A., & Wilber, C. (1984). Psychodynamic theories of opiate addiction: New directions for research. *Clinical Psychology Review, 4*, 159-189.

Blatt, S. J., Rounsaville, B., Eyre, S. L., & Wilber, C. (1984). The psychodynamics of opiate addiction. *The Journal of Nervous and Mental Disease*, 172(6), 342-352.

Blatt, S. J., Quinlan, D.M., Chevron, E., McDonald, C., & Zuroff, D. (1982). Dependency and self-criticism: Psychological dimensions of depression. *Journal of Consulting and Clinical Psychology, 50*, 113-124.

Borg, W. R., & Gall, M. D. (1983). *Educational research: An introduction*. New York, NY: Longman.

Boyer, L. B. (1978). On the mutual influences of anthropology and psychoanalysis. *Journal of Psychological Anthropology, 1*, 265-296.

Boyer, L. B. (1979a). Countertransference with severely regressed patients. In Epstein, L., & Feiner, A. H. (Eds.). *Countertransference: The therapist's contribution to the therapeutic situation*. Northvale, NJ: Jason Aronson.

Boyer, L.B. (1979b). *Childhood and folklore: A psychoanalytic study of Apache personality*. New York, NY: Library of Psychological Anthropology.

Boyer, L. B. (1983). *The regressed patient*. Northvale, NJ: Jason Aronson.

Boyer, L. B. (1992). *Countertransference: Brief history and clinical issues with regressed patients.* Presented at the Center for the Advanced Study of the Psychoses, San Francisco, CA.

Boyer, L. B., Boyer, R. M., Dithrich, C. W., Harned, H., Hippler, A. E., Stone, J. S., & Walt, A. (1989). The relation between psychological states and acculturation among the Tanaina and Upper Tanana Indians of Alaska. *Ethos, 17,* 387-427.

Boyer, L. B. & Giovacchini, P. L. (Eds.). (1990). *Master Clinicians on treating the regressed patient. Vol. 1.* Northvale, NJ: Jason Aronson.

Boyer, L. B. & Giovacchini, P. L. (Eds.). (1993). *Master Clinicians on treating the regressed patient. Vol. 2.* Northvale, NJ: Jason Aronson.

Brill, L. (1977). The treatment of drug abuse: Evolution of a perspective. *American Journal of Psychiatry, 134*(2), 157-160.

Brink, A. (1985). Bertrand Russell: The angry pacifist. *Journal of Psychohistory, 12*(4), 497-514.

Brook, J. S., Whiteman, M., Scovell, A., & Brenden, C. (1983). Older brother's influence on younger sibling's drug use. *The Journal of Psychology, 114,* 83-90.

Bry, B., McKeon, P., & Pandrina, R. J. (1982). Extent of drug use as a number of risk factors. *Journal of Abnormal Psychology, 91,* 273-279.

Buckley, P. (1986). *Essential papers on object relations.* New York, NY: New York University press.

Callea, G., & Rubino, A. I. (1980). Appunti sull'incidenza e la struttura dei disturbi della personalita [Some notes on the incidence and structure of personality disorders]. *Lavoro Neuropsichiatrico, 67*(3), 255-263.

Campbell, D. T., & Stanley, J.C. (1963). *Experimental and quasi-experimental designs for research.* New York, NY: Houghton Mifflen Company.

Cashdan, S. (1988). *Object relations therapy: Using the relationship.* New York, NY: W. W. Norton & Co.

Charles-Nicolas, A., Valleur, M., & Tonnelier, H. (1982). Enfance et Drogue [Childhood and Drugs]. *Psychiatrie de l'Enfant,* 25(1), 207-253.

Chasnoff, J. J. (1987). Perinatal effects of cocaine. *Contemporary Obstetrics and Gynecology, 29*(5), 163-179.

Chatlos, C. (1987). *Crack: What you should know about the cocaine epidemic.* New York, NY: Perigee Books.

Chessick, R. D. (1983). Marilyn Monroe: Psychoanalytic pathography of a preoedipal disorder. *Psychoanalysis, 72,* 1367.

Ciambelli, M., & Portanova, F. (1980). Psicoanalisi e arte: Il problema dell'interpretazione [Psychoanalysis and art: The problem of interpretation]. *Psicologia e Societa, 3,* 30-32.

Clerici, M., Capitano, C., Poterzio, F., Ba, G., et al. (1986). Toxicomanie et regression narcissique etudiees dans la relation medicament-patient [Drug addiction and narcissistic regression studied in the patient-medicine relationship]. *Psychologie-Medicale, 18*(2), 279-281.

Coombs, R. H., Fawzy, F. I., & Gerber, B. E. (1984). Patterns of substance use among adolescents: A longitudinal study. *Substance and Alcohol Actions/Misuse, 5,* 59-67.

Cotten, L. (1985). *All shook up: Elvis day-by-day, 1954-1977.* Ann Arbor, MI: Pierian Press.

DeAngelis, G. G. (1975). Theoretical and clinical approaches to the treatment of drug addiction: With special considerations for the adolescent drug abuser. *Journal of Psychedelic Drugs, 7*(2), 187-202.

Deutsch, H. (1982). George Sand: A woman's destiny. *International Review of Psychoanalysis, 9*(4), 445-460.

DeVos, G. A. & Boyer, L. B. (1989). *Symbolic analysis cross-culturally: The Roschach Test*. Berkeley, CA: The University of California Press.

Dielhman, T. E., Campanelli, P. C., Shope, J. T., & Buchart, A. T. (1987). Susceptibility to peer pressure, self-esteem, and health locus of control as correlates of adolescent substance abuse. *Health Education Quarterly, 14*(2), 207-221.

Dodes, L. M. (1990). Addiction, helplessness, and narcissistic rage. *The Psychoanalytic Quarterly, 59*(3), 398-419.

Dorpat, T. L. (1976). Structural conflict and object relations conflict. *Journal of the American Psychoanalytical Association, 24*, 855-874.

Duncan, D. F. (1987). Cocaine smoking and its implication for health and health education. *Health Education, 18*(4), 24-27.

Dubosc-Benabou, I. (1990). Dionysos ou les advantages et les inconvenients de la diversite [Dionysus, or the pros and cons of mutlifariousness]. *Psychanalyse a l'Universite, 15*(58), 67-84.

Edelson, M. (1988). *Psychoanalysis: A theory in crisis*. Chicago, IL: University of Chicago Press.

Edelstein, E. L. (1975). Elaborations on the meaning of repetitive behavior in drug dependent personalities. *British Journal of Addiction, 70*, 365-373.

Emde, R. (1983). The prepresentational self and its affective care. *The Psychoanalytic Study of the Child, 38*, 165-192.

Ensminger, M. E., Brown, H., & Kellam, S. G. (1982). Sex difference in antecedents of substance abuse among adolescents. *Journal of Social Issues, 38,* 25-42.

Erikson, E. H. (1956). The problem of ego identity. *The Journal of the American Psychoanalytical Association, 4,* 56-121.

Euripides. (1954). *The Bacchae and other plays.* Middlesex, England: Penquin Books.

Fairbairn, W. H. D. (1952). *Psychoanalytic studies of the personality.* London, England: Routledge & Kegan Paul, Ltd.

Falco, M. (1988). *Preventing abuse of drugs, alcohol and tobacco by adolescents.* Washington, DC: Carnegie Council on Adolescent Development.

Federn, P. (1952). *Ego psychology and the psychoses.* New York, NY: Basic Books.

Fenichel, O. (1945). *The psychoanalytic theory of neurosis.* New York, NY: Norton.

Fine, R. (1972). The psychoanalysis of a drug addict. *The Psychoanalytic Review, 59*(4), 585-608.

Fisher, S., & Greenberg, R. P. (1985). The scientific credibility of Freud's theories and therapy. New York, NY: Columbia University Press.

Freud, A. (1946). *The Psycho-analytical treatment of children.* New York, NY: International Universities Press.

Freud, S. (1900). The interpretation of dreams. In the *Standard Edition of the Complete Psychological Works of Sigmund Freud* (Vols. 4–5). London, England: Hogarth Press.

Freud, S. (1910). Leonardo da Vinci and memory of his childhood. In the *Standard Edition of the Complete Psychological Works of Sigmund Freud* (Vol. 11). London, England: The Hogarth Press.

Freud, S. (1917). Mourning and melancholia. In the *Standard Edition of the Complete Psychological Works of Sigmund Freud* (Vol. 14). London, England: The Hogarth Press.

Freud, S. (1920). Beyond the pleasure principle. In the *Standard Edition of the Complete Psychological Works of Sigmund Freud* (Vol. 18). London, England: The Hogarth Press.

Freud, S. (1926). Inhibitions, symptoms and anxiety. In the *Standard Edition of the Complete Psychological Works of Sigmund Freud* (Vol. 20). London, England: The Hogarth Press.

Freud, S. (1927). Fetishism. In the *Standard Edition of the Complete Psychological Works of Sigmund Freud* (Vol. 21). London, England: The Hogarth Press.

Freud, S. (1928). Dostoevsky and parricide. In the *Standard Edition of the Complete Psychological Works of Sigmund Freud* (Vol. 21). London, England: The Hogarth Press.

Freud, S. (1933). New introductory lectures on psychoanalysis. In the *Standard Edition of the Complete Psychological Works of Sigmund Freud* (Vol. 22). London, England: The Hogarth Press.

Freud, S. (1939). Moses and Monotheism. In the *Standard Edition of the Complete Psychological Works of Sigmund Freud* (Vol. 23). London, England: The Hogarth Press.

Freud, S. (1985). *The complete letters of Sigmund Freud to Wilhem Fliess.* Cambridge, MA: Harvard University Press.

Furman, B. (1986). On trauma: When is the death of a parent traumatic. *Psychoanalytic Study of the Child, 41,* 191-208.

Gayda, M., & Vacola, G. (1988). Initiation et hysterie [Initiation and hysteria]. *Psychiatrie Francaise*, 19, 87-90.

Giorgi, A. (1970). *Psychology as a human science.* New York, NY: Harper and Row.

Giovacchini, P. L. (1989). *Countertransference: Triumphs and Catastrophes.* Northvale, NJ: Jason Aronson.

Ghaffari, K. (1987). Psycho analytic theories on drug dependence: A critical review. *Psychoanalytic Psychotherapy*, 3(1), 39-51.

Glover, E. (1939). *Psychoanalysis, 2nd Edition.* London, England: Staple Press.

Gottesfeld, M. L., Caroff, P., & Lieberman, F. (1973). Treatment of adolescent drug abusers. *Psychoanalytic Review*, 59(4), 527-537.

Greaves, G. B. (1980). An existential theory of drug dependence. In D. J. Lettieri, M. Sayers, & H. W. Pearson (Eds.). *Theories on drug use: Selected contemporary perspectives.* (GPO Stock Number 017-024-00997). Washington, DC: U.S. Government Printing Office.

Green, A. (1986). *On private madness.* London, England: Hogarth Press.

Greenacre, P. (1969). The fetish and the transitional object. *Psychoanalytic Study of the Child*, 24, 144-164.

Greenacre, P. (1970). The transitional object and the fetish with special reference to the role of illusion. *International Journal of Psychoanalysis*, 51, 447-456.

Greenspan, S. (1989). *The development of the ego: Implications for personality theory, psychopathology, and the psychotherapeutic process.* Madison, CT: International Universities press.

Grenier, C. (1985). Treatment effectiveness in an adolescent chemical dependency treatment program: A quasi-experimental design. *International Journal of the Addictions, 20*(3), 381-391.

Grof, S. (1973). Theoretical and empirical basis of transpersonal psychotherapy. *Journal of Transpersonal Psychology, 5,* 15-53.

Grof, S. (1985). Modern consciousness research and human survival. Ninth conference of the International Transpersonal Association. *ReVISION, 8*(1), 27-39.

Haas, A. P. (1987). Long-term outcomes of heavy marijuana use among adolescents. *Drug and Alcohol use in Children and Adolescence: Pediatrician, 14,* 77-82.

Hamilton, E. (1940). *Mythology.* New York, NY: Basic Books.

Hammontree, P. G. (1985). *Elvis Presley: A bio-bibliography.* Westport, CT: Greenwood Press.

Hartmann, D. (1969). A study of drug taking adolescents. *The Psychoanalytic Study of the Child, 24,* 384-398.

Hartmann, H. (1952). The mutual influences in the development of the Ego and Id. *The Psychoanalytic Study of the Child, 7,* 7-17.

Hawkins, J. D., Jenson, J. M., Catalano, R. F., & Lishner, D. M. (1988). Delinquency and drug abuse: Implications for social services. *Social Services review, 62*(2), 258-284.

Hawkins, J. D., Lishner, D. M., & Catalano, R. F. (1986). Childhood predictors and the prevention of adolescent substance abuse. In C. L. Jones & R. J. Battjes (Eds.). *Etiology of drug abuse: Implications for prevention.* (DHHS Publication Number ADM85-1385). Washington, DC: National Institute of Drug Abuse.

Hawkins, J. D., Lishner, D. M., Catalano, R. F., & Howard, M. O. (1986). Childhood predictors and the prevention of adolescent substance abuse: Toward an empirically grounded theory. *Journal of Children in Contemporary Society, 8*(1), 11-48.

Henderson, D. (1981). '*Skuse me while I kiss the sky: The life of Jimi Hendrix*. New York, NY: Bantam Books.

Hoffer, W. (1955). *Psychoanalysis: Practical and research aspects*. Baltimore, MD: Williams and Wilkins.

Horan, J. J., & Williams, J. M. (1982). Longitudinal study of assertion training as a drug abuse prevention strategy. *American Educational Research Journal, 19*(3), 341-351.

Hundleby, J. D., & Mercer, G. W. (1987). Family and friends as social environments and their relationship to young adolescents' use of alcohol, tobacco, and marijuana. *Journal of Marriage and Family, 49*, 151-164.

Inciardi, J. A. (1991). (Ed.). *The drug legalization debate*. Beverly Hills, CA: Sage Publications.

Jacobsen, E. (1964). *The self and the object world*. New York, NY: International Universities Press.

Jessor, R. (1979). Marijuana: A review of recent psychosocial research. In R. Dupont, A. Goldstein, & J. O'Donnell (Eds.). *Handbook on drug abuse*. Washington, DC: National Institute of Drug Abuse.

Jessor, R., Jessor, S. L., & Finney, J. (1973). A social psychology of marijuana use: Longitudinal studies of high school and college youth. *Journal of Personality and Social Psychology, 26*, 1-15.

Johnson, G. M., Shontz, F. C., & Locke, T. P. (1984). Relationships between adolescent drug use and parental drug behaviors. *Adolescence, 14*(74), 296-299.

Johnston, L. D., O'Malley, P. M., & Bachman, J. G. (1987). *National trends in drug use and related factors among American high school students and young adults, 1975-1986.* (DHHS Publication number ADM87-1535). Rockville, MD: National Institute of Drug Abuse.

Institute of Medicine. (1982). *Marijuana and health.* Washington, DC: National Academy Press.

Jones, J. (1961). *The life and work of Sigmund Freud.* New York, NY: Basic Books.

Kandel, D. B. (1975). Adolescent marijuana use: Role of parents and peers. *Science, 181,* 1067-1070.

Kandel, D. B. (1980). Drug and drinking behavior among youth. *Annual Review of Sociology, 6,* 235-285.

Kandel, D. B., & Adler, I. (1982). Socialization into marijuana use among French adolescents: A cross-cultural comparison with the United States. *Journal of Health and Social Behavior, 23,* 295-309.

Kandel, D. B., & Faust, R. (1975). Sequence and stages of patterns of adolescent drug use. *Archives of General Psychiatry, 32,* 923-932.

Kandel, D. B., & Logan J. A. (1984). Patterns of drug use from adolescence to young adulthood: Period of risk for initiation, continued use, and discontinuance. *American Journal of Public Health, 74,* 660-666.

Kandel, D. B., Kessler, R., & Margulies, R. (1978). Antecedents of adolescent initiation into drug stages of drug use: A developmental analysis. *Journal of Youth and Adolescence, 7,* 13-40.

Katan, A. (1973). Children who were raped. *Psychoanalytic Study of the Child, 28,* 208-224.

Kerényi, C. (1951). *The gods of the Greeks*. New York, NY: Thames and Hudson.

Kernberg, O. F. (1967). Borderline personality organization. *Journal of the American Psychoanalytical Association, 13*, 38-56.

Kernberg, O. F. (1975). *Borderline conditions and pathological narcissism*. New York, NY: Jason Aronson.

Kernberg, O. F. (1976). Forword to V. D. Volkan, *Primitive internalized object relations*. New York, NY: International Universities Press.

Kernberg, O. F. (1980). *Internal world and external reality: Object relations theory applied*. New York, NY: Jason Aronson.

Kernberg, O. F. (1984). *Severe personality disorders: Psychotherapeutic strategies*. New Haven, CT: Yale University Press.

Kernberg, P. (1989). Narcissistic personality disorder in childhood. *The Psychiatric Clinics of North America, 12*, 671-694.

Kestenberg, J. S., & Brenner, I. (1985). *Children who survived the Holocaust: The roles and routines in the development of the superego*. Paper presented at the 34th Congress of the International Psychoanalytic Association, Hamburg, Germany.

Keyes, S., & Block, J. (1984). Prevalence and patterns of substance use among early adolescents. *Journal of Youth and Adolescence, 13*(1), 1-15.

Khantzian, E. J. (1972). A preliminary dynamic formulation of the psychopharmacologic action of methadone. *Proceedings of the Fourth National Methadone Conference*, San Francisco, CA.

Khantzian, E. J. (1974). Opiate addiction: A critique of theory and some implications for treatment. *American Journal of Psychotherapy, 28,* 59-70.

Khantzian, E. J. (1975). Self selection and progression in drug dependence. *Psychiatry Digest, 10,* 19-22.

Khantzian, E. J. (1978). The ego, the self and opiate addiction: Theoretical and treatment considerations. *International Review of Psychoanalysis, 5,*189-198.

Khantzian, E. J. (1979). Impulse problems in addiction: cause and effect relationships. In Wishnie, H. (Ed.). *Working with the Impulsive Person.* New York, NY: Plenum Publishing.

Khantzian, E. J. (1980). An ego-self theory of substance dependence. In Lettieri, D. J., Sayars, M., & Wallenstein, H. W. (Eds.). *Theories of Addiction. NIDA Monograph #30.* Rockville, MD: National Institute on Drug Abuse.

Khantzian, E. J. (1982). Psychological (structural) vulnerabilities and the specific appeal of narcotics. *Annals of the New York Academy of Sciences, 398,* 24-32.

Khantzian, E. J. (1985). The self-medication hypothesis of addictive disorders. *American Journal of Psychiatry, 142*(11), 1259-1264.

Khantzian, E. J. (1987a). A clinical perspective of the cause-consequence controversy in alcoholic and addictive suffering. *Journal of the American Academy of Psychoanalysis, 15,* 512-537.

Khantzian, E. J. (1987b). *Substance dependence, repetition and the nature of addictive suffering.* Presented at the 76th Annual Meeting of the American Psychoanalytic Association, Chicago, IL.

Khantzian, E. J. (1989). Addiction: Self-Destruction or Self-Repair? *Journal of Substance Abuse Treatment, 6,* 75.

Khantzian, E. J. (1990). *Self-regulation vulnerabilities in substance abusers: Treatment implications.* Paper presented at the American Psychoanalytic Association Workshop for Clinicians, November.

Khantzian, E. J. & Kates, W. W. (1978). Group treatment of unwilling addicted patients: programmatic and clinical aspects. *International Journal of Group Psychotherapy, 1*(1), 81-94.

Khantzian, E. J. & Treece, C. (1977). Psychodynamics of drug dependence: An overview. In Blaine, J. D. & Julius, D. A. (Eds.). *Psychodynamics of Drug Dependence. NIDA Monograph #12.* Rockville, MD: National Institute on Drug Abuse.

Klein, M. (1959). *The psycho-analysis of children.* London, England: The Hogarth Press LTD.

Knight, R. P. (1938). The psychoanalytic treatment in a sanitarium of chronic addiction to alcohol. *Journal of the American Medical Association*, 111.

Kohut, H. (1971). *The analysis of the self: A systematic approach to the psychoanalytic treatment of narcissistic personality disorders.* New York, NY: International Universities Press.

Kohut, H. (1977). *The restoration of the self.* New York, NY: International Universities Press.

Kohut, H. (1978). Thoughts on narcissism and narcissistic rage. In Ornstein, P. H. (Ed.). *The search for the self.* New York, NY: International Universities Press.

Kohut, H. (1984). *How does analysis cure?* Chicago, IL: University of Chicago Press.

Kramer, E. (1971). *Art therapy with children.* New York, NY: Schocken Books.

Krys, E. (1952). *Psychoanalytic explorations in art.* New York, NY: Schoken Books.

Krystal, H. (1977). Aspects of affect theory. *Bulletin of the Menninger Clinic, 41*(1), 1-26.

Krystal, H. & Raskin, H. A. (1970). *Drug dependence: Aspects of ego functions.* Detroit, MI: Wayne State University Press.

Lacan, J. (1982). *Feminine sexuality.* New York, NY: W. W. Norton & Company.

Lagache, D. (1966). Psychoanalysis as an exact science. In Lowenstein, R. M., Newman, L. M., Schur, M., & Solnit, A. J. (Eds.). *Psychoanalysis as a general psychology: Essays in honor of Heinz Hartmann.* New York, NY: International Universities Press.

Langs, R. (1976). The misalliance dimension in Freud's case histories: I. The case of Dora. *International Journal of Psychoanalytic Psychotherapy, 5,* 301-317.

Lawton, H. W. (1990). The field of psychohistory. *Journal of Psychohistory, 17*(4), 353-364.

Lee, M. A., & Shlain, B. (1985). *Acid dreams: The CIA, LSD and the sixties rebellion.* New York, NY: Grove Press.

Levin, J. D. (1987). *Treatment of alcoholism and other addictions: A self-psychology approach.* Northvale, NJ: Jason Aronson Inc.

Lidz, T., Lidz, R. W., & Rubenstein, R. (1976). An anaclitic syndrome in adolescent amphetamine addicts. *Psychoanalytic Study of the Child, 31,* 317-348.

Lifton, R. J. (1968). *Revolutionary immortality: Mao Tse-tung and the Chinese Cultural Revolution.* New York, NY: Random House.

Ling, T. M., & Buckman, J. (1965). The treatment of frigidity with LSD & Ritalin. In Weil, G. M., Metzner, R., & Leary, T. (Eds.). *The psychedelic reader.* New Hyde Park, NY: University Books, Inc.

Lowenfeld, M. (1979). *The world technique.* London, England: George Allen & Unwin.

Luzzatto, P. (1987). The internal world of drug-abusers: Projective pictures of self-object relationships: A pilot study. *British Journal of Projective Psychology, 32*(2), 22-33.

Mahler, M. S. (1968). *On human symbiosis and the vicissitudes of individuation.* New York, NY: International Universities Press.

Mahler, M. S., Pine, F., & Bergman, A. (1975). *The psychological birth of the human infant: Symbiosis and individuation.* New York, NY: Basic Books.

Mahon, E. J. (1987). Ancient mariner, Pilot's boy: A Note on the creativity of Samuel Coleridge. *Psychoanalytic Study of the Child, 42,* 489-509.

Marcos, A. C., & Bahr, S. J. (1988). Control theory and adolescent drug use. *Youth and Society, 19*(4), 395-425.

Martin, J. (1983). William Faulkner: Construction and reconstruction in biography and psychoanalysis. *Psychoanalytic Inquiry, 3*(2), 295-340.

McDermott, J. (1992). *Hendrix: Setting the record straight.* New York, NY: Warner Books, Inc.

McDougall, J. (1984). The dis-affected patient: Reflections on affect pathology. *Psychoanalytic Quarterly, 53,* 386-409.

McDougall, J. (1985). *Theaters of the mind: Illusion and truth on the psychoanalytic stage.* New York, NY: Basic Books.

McLellan, A. T., Woody, G.E., & O'Brien, C. P. (1979). Development of psychiatric illness in drug abusers: Possible role of drug preference. *New England Journal of Medicine, 310*, 1310-1313.

McVay, D. (1991). Marijuana legalization: The time is now. In Inciardi, J. A. (Ed.). *The drug legalization debate.* Beverly Hills, CA: Sage Publications.

Meadow, P. W. (1984). Issues in psychoanalytic research. *Modern Psychoanalysis, 9*(2), 123-147.

Meeks, J. (1985). Adolescents at risk for drug and alcohol abuse. *Seminars in Adolescent Medicine, 1*(14), 231-233.

Mider, P. A. (1983). Personality typologies of addicts by drug of choice. *Bulletin of the Society of Psychologists in Addictive Behaviors, 2*(3), 197-217.

Mijuskovic, B. (1988). Loneliness and adolescent alcoholism. *Adolescence, 23*(91), 504-516.

Miller, P. (1983). Se faire la peau (1) [Growing a skin: 1.]. *Topique Revue Freudienne, 13*(31), 51-91.

Mitchell, J. (1982). Introduction I. In Lacan, J. *Feminine sexuality.* New York, NY: W. W. Norton and Company.

Moskowitz, J. M. (1983). Preventing adolescent substance abuse through education. In T. J. Glynn, C. G. Leukfeld, & J. P. Ludford (Eds.) *Preventing adolescent drug abuse:* · *Intervention strategies* (p. 233-249). (NTIS Pub. No. 85-159663/AS). Washington, DC: U.S. Government Printing Office.

Nadelmann, E. A. (1989, September). Drug prohibition in the United States: Costs, consequences, and alternatives. *Science, 245*, 939-947.

Naumberg, M. (1973). *An introduction to art therapy: Studies of the 'free' art expression of behavior problem children and adolescents as a means of diagnosis and therapy*. New York, NY: Teachers College Press.

Newcomb, M. D., & Harlow, L. L. (1986). Life events and substance use among adolescents: Mediating effects of perceived loss of control and meaninglessness in life. *Journal of Personality and Social Psychology, 51*(3), 564-577.

Newcomb, M. D., Maddhian, E., & Bentler, P. M. (1986). Risk factors for drug use among adolescents: Concurrent and longitudinal analyses. *American Journal of Public health, 76,* 525-531.

Panken, S. (1983). "Working through" and the novel. *Psychoanalytic Review, 70*(1), 4-23.

Perry, C. L., & Murray, D. M. (1985). The prevention of adolescent drug abuse: Implications from etiological, developmental and environmental models. *Journal of Primary Prevention, 6*(1), 31-52.

Peterson, R. C. (1984). Marijuana overview, In M. D. Glantz (Ed.). *Correlates of marijuana use*. Rockville, MD: National Institute of Drug Abuse.

Pickens, K. (1985). Drug education: The effects of giving information. *Journal of Alcohol and Drug Education, 30*(3), 32-44.

Pollock, G. H. (1986). Oedipus examined and reconsidered: The myth, the developmental stage, the universal theme, the conflict, and the complex. *Annual of Psychoanalysis, 14,* 77-106.

Rabow, J. (1983). Psychoanalysis and social science: A review. *Psychohistory Review, 12*(1), 34-41.

Radford, P.T., Wiseberg, S., & Yorke, C. (1971). A study of "main-line" heroin addiction: A preliminary report. *Psychoanalytic Study of the Child, 27,* 156-180.

Rado, S. (1933). Psychoanalysis of Pharmacothymia. *Psychoanalytic Quarterly, 2,* 1-23.

Ravenholt, R. T. (1984). Addictive mortality in the United States 1980: Tobacco, alcohol and other substances. *Population Development Review, 10,* 697-724.

Romanyshyn, R. D. (1978). Psychology and the attitude of science. In Valle, R. S., & King, M. (Eds.). *Existential-phenomenological alternatives for psychology.* New York, NY: Oxford University Press.

Rosenbaum, M., & Doblin, R. (1990). Why MDMA should not have been made illegal. In Inciardi, J. A. (Ed.). *The drug legalization debate.* Beverly Hills, CA: Sage Publications.

Rosenfeld, H. A. (1965). *Psychotic States.* New York, NY: International Universities Press.

Rosenfeld, D. A. (1976). *Clinica psicoanalîtica estudios sobre drogadiccion, psicosis y narcisismo.* Buenos Aires, Argentina: Editorial Galerna.

Rosenfeld, D. A. (1992). *The psychotic: Aspects of the personality.* London, UK: Karnac Books.

Rosenfeld, D. A. (1993). Drug abuse, regression, and primitive object relations. In Boyer, L. B. & Giovaochini, P. L. (Eds.). *Master clinicians on treating the regressed patient. Vol. 2.* Northvale, NJ: Jason Aronson.

Rosenman, S. (1988). The myth of the birth of the hero revisisted: Disasters and brutal child rearing. *American Imago, 45*(1), 1-44.

Runyan, W. M. (1980). In defense of the case study method. *American Journal of Orthopsychiatry, 52*(3), 440-446.

Sarnoff, I. (1971). *Testing Freudian concepts: An experimental social approach.* New York, NY: Springer Publications.

Savitt, R. A. (1954). Extramural psychoanalytic treatment of a case of narcotic addiction. *Journal of the American Psychoanalytic Association, 2,* 494-502.

Schiffer, F. (1988). Psychotherapy of nine successfully treated cocaine abusers: Techniques and dynamics. *Journal of Substance Abuse Treatment, 5,* 131-137.

Searles, H. F. (1986). *My work with borderline patients.* Northvale, NJ: Jason Aronson.

Segal, B. (1986). Intervention and prevention of drug taking behavior: A need for divergent approaches. *International Journal of Addictions, 21,* 165-173.

Seymor, R. B., & Smith, D. E. (1987). *Drugfree: A unique positive approach to staying off alcohol and other drugs.* New York, NY: Sarah Lazin Books.

Shapiro, H., & Glebbeek, C. (1990). *Jimi Hendrix: Electric gypsy.* New York, NY: St. Martin's Press.

Shedler, J., & Block, J. (1990). Adolescent drug use and psychological health: A longitudinal inquiry. *American Psychologist, 45*(5), 612-630.

Smith, D. E. (1970). (Ed.). *The new social drug: Cultural, medical and legal perspectives on marijuana.* Englewood Cliffs, NJ: Prentice-Hall, Inc.

Smith, R. C. (1968). U. S. marijuana legislation and the creation of a social problem. *Journal of Psychedelic Drugs, 2*(1), 93-103.

Smith, T., Koob, J., & Wirtz, T. (1985). Ecology of adolescents' marijuana abuse. *The International Journal of Addictions, 20*(9), 1421-1428.

Socarides, C. W. (1968). *The overt homosexual.* New York, NY: Grune and Stratton.

Socarides, C. W. (1974). Homosexuality. In Arieti, S. (Ed.). *American handbook of psychiatry; 2nd edition*. New York, NY: Basic Books.

Socarides, C. W. (1985). Depression in perversion: With special reference to the function of erotic experience in sexual perversion. In Volkan, V.D. (Ed.). *Depressive states and their treatment*. Northvale, NJ: Jason Aronson.

Spitz, E. H. (1985). *Art and psyche: A study in psychoanalysis and aesthetics*. New Haven, CT: Yale University Press.

Sptiz, E. H. (1987). Separation-individuation in a cycle of songs: George Crumb's Ancient Voices of Children. *The Psychoanalytic Study of the Child, 42*, 531-543.

Spitz, E. H. (1991). *Museums of the mind*. Paper presented at The Conference on Psychoanalysis and Culture: Contributions of Sigmund Freud, Stanford University, January 13.

Spitz, R. A. (1946). Anaclitic depression. *The Psychoanalytic Study of Children, 2*, 313-342.

Statistical Bulletin. (1984). *Drinking and driving, 65*(3), 2-7.

Stern, D. N. (1985). *The interpersonal world of the infant*. New York, NY: Basic Books.

Surgeon General. (1979). *Smoking and health: A report to the Surgeon General*. (DHEW Publication Number PHS79-50066). Washington, DC: U.S. Government Printing Office.

Sutton, L. R. (1983). The effects of alcohol, marijuana and their combination on driving ability. *Journal of Studies on Alcohol, 44*(3), 438-445.

Symington, N. (1986). *The Analytic Experience*. New York, NY: St. Martin's Press.

Szasz, T. S. (1992). *Our right to drugs: The case for a free market.* Westport, CT: Greenwood Publishers.

Tähkä, V. (1988). On the early formation of the mind, II: From differentiation to self and object constancy. *The Psychoanalytic Study of the Child, 43,* 101-134.

Thorne, C. R., & Deblassie, R. R. (1985). Adolescent substance abuse. *Adolescence, 20*(78), 335-347.

Trepper, T. S. (1990). In celebration of the case study. *Journal of Family Psychotherapy, 1*(1), 5-13.

Trevisano, M. A. (1990). *Compensatory object choice in children and adults with histories of maternal deprivation.* Unpublished doctoral dissertation. Center for Psychological Studies, Albany CA.

Ulman, E., & Dachinger, P. (Eds.). (1975). *Art therapy in theory and practice.* New York, NY: Schocken Books.

Valle, R. S., & King, M. (Eds.) (1978). *Existential-phenomenological alternatives for psychology.* New York, NY: Oxford University Press.

Villoldo, A. (1977). An introduction to the psychedelic psychotherapy of Salvador Roquet. *Journal of Humanistic Psychology, 17*(4), 45-58.

Volkan, K. (1991). *Drug Use and Object Relations Theory: An Integration of Fairbairn's Theory and the Classical Drive/Structure Model.* Presented at the California Psychological Association Annual Convention, February 22, San Diego, CA.

Volkan, K., & Fetro, J. V. (1990). Substance use prevention: Implications of theory and practice for school-based programs. *Family Life Educator, 8*(4), 17-23.

Volkan, V. D. (1976). *Primitive internalized object relations.* New York, NY: International Universities Press.

Volkan, V. D. (1979). *Cyprus—war and adaptation: A psychoanalytic history of two ethnic groups in conflict.* Charlottesville, VA: University of Virginia Press.

Volkan, V. D. (1981). *Linking objects and linking phenomena.* New York, NY: International Universities Press.

Volkan, V. D. (1987). *Six steps in the treatment of borderline personality organization.* Northvale, NJ: Jason Aronson.

Volkan, V. D. (1988). *A discussion of the "Genesis of Perversions: The Development of a Fetish" by George Zavitzianos.* Annual Meeting of the American Psychoanalytic Association, Montreal, Canada, May 4 -8.

Volkan, V. D., & Itzkowitz, N. (1984). *The immortal Atatürk: A psychobiography.* Chicago, IL: University of Chicago Press.

Volkan, V. D., & Kavanaugh, J. (1988). The cat people. In Grolnick, S. A., & Barkin, L. (Eds.). *Between Reality and Fantasy.* Northvale, NJ: Jason Aronson.

Wallack, L., Corbett, K. (1987). Alcohol, tobacco and marijuana use among youth: An overview of epidemiological program and policy trends. *Health Education Quarterly, 14*(2), 223-249.

Wasserman, D., & Cullberg, J. (1989). Early separation and suicidal behavior in the parental homes of 40 consecutive suicide attempters. *Acta Psychiatrica Scandinavica, 79*(3), 296-302.

Weider, H. & Kaplan, E. (1969). Drug use in adolescents. *Psychoanalytic Study of the Child, 24,* 399-431.

Weil, A. T., & Rosen, W. (1983). *Chocolate to Morphine: Understanding mind active drugs.* Boston, MA: Houghton Mifflin Co.

Winnicott, D. W. (1951). Transitional objects and transitional phenomena. In *Collected papers*. New York, NY: Basic Books.

Winnicott, D. W. (1989). *Psycho-Analytic explorations*. Cambridge, MA: Harvard University Press.

Wurmser, L. (1974). Psychoanalytic considerations of the etiology of compulsive drug use. *Journal of the American Psychoanalytical Association, 22* 820-843.

Wurmser, L. (1978). *The hidden dimension: Psychodynamics in compulsive drug use.* New York, NY: Jason Aronson.

Wurmser, L. (1985). Denial and split identity: Timely issues in the psychoanalytic psychotherapy of compulsive drug users. *Journal of Substance Abuse Treatment, 2,* 89-96.

Wurmser, L. (1987). Flight from conscience: Experiences with the psychoanalytic treatment of compulsive drug abusers. *Journal of Substance Abuse Treatment, 4,* 157-168.

Yamaguchi, K., & Kandel, D. B. (1984a). Patterns of drug use from adolescence to young adulthood: Sequences of progression. *American Journal of Public Health, 74,* 668-672.

Yamaguchi, K., & Kandel, D. B. (1984b). Patterns of drug use from adolescence to young adulthood: Predictors of progression. *American Journal of Public Health, 74,* 673-681.

Zinberg, N. E. (1975). Addiction and ego functions. *Psychoanalytic Study of the Child, 30,* 567-588.

Index

Abadi, 26
Abraham, 25, 27
  alcohol use, 27
  alcoholism, 27
  character formation, 27
  drinking in a bar, 27
  homosexuality, 28
  infantile oral state, 28
  oral conflicts, 27
  psychosexual phases, 27
abstinence, 119
abuse, 10
accidental deaths, 71
Acid Dreams, 8
acting out, 36, 75, 93, 94
Adams-Silvan & Adams, 82
adaptive mechanisms, 40
addict, 31, 36
addict lacking a skin, 39
addiction, 10, 30
addictive object, 63
Adler, 52
admission of addiction, 116
adolescence, 20, 21, 22, 103, 104
  alcohol, 20
  cigarette smoking, 20
  high school students, 20

illegal drugs other than marijuana, 20
affect, 40, 47, 48, 50, 57, 75
aggression, 27, 48, 59, 69
aggressive drive, 29, 35, 47, 57, 65
Alaska, 8
alcohol, 7, 13, 20, 21, 49, 63, 124
alcohol dependence, 13
alcoholics, 45
Alcoholics Anonymous, 116
all-powerful mother figure, 100
Almansi, 81
altered state of consciousness, 41
America, 15, 113
American Medical Association, 123
American Psychiatric Association, 9
amphetamine abusers, 14, 75, 101, 109
amphetamine use, 14
amphetamines, 14, 75, 98, 101, 103
anaclitic depression, 43, 44, 104

The Reshaping of Psychoanalysis
From Sigmund Freud to Ernest Becker

This series is designed to offer works which are concerned with the reshaping and revitalization of psychoanalysis. Also critical to this series is the interweaving of such disciplines as psychology, psychiatry, religion, and philosophy so as to promote dialogue and offer avenues toward rapprochement.

This series will publish and proffer studies of Freud and Neo-Freudians such as Becker which are most aware of the long term contributions of psychoanalysis toward the healing of self and society. Studies should be scholarly and clinically discerning. This is a series which is keenly concerned with the bridging of disciplines, the networking of ideas and peoples, and with the perpetuation of the psychoanalytic questions, and, at times, its answers. This is a series which is also very open to its authors' creativity and most appreciative of those efforts which reshape, revamp, revitalize, and transform Freudian psychoanalysis.

The General Series Editor is Barry R. Arnold, an Emory Ph.D., who is Associate Professor of Religious Studies and Philosophy at the University of West Florida. His speciality area is psychoanalysis and medical ethics.